Finding
N·E·D

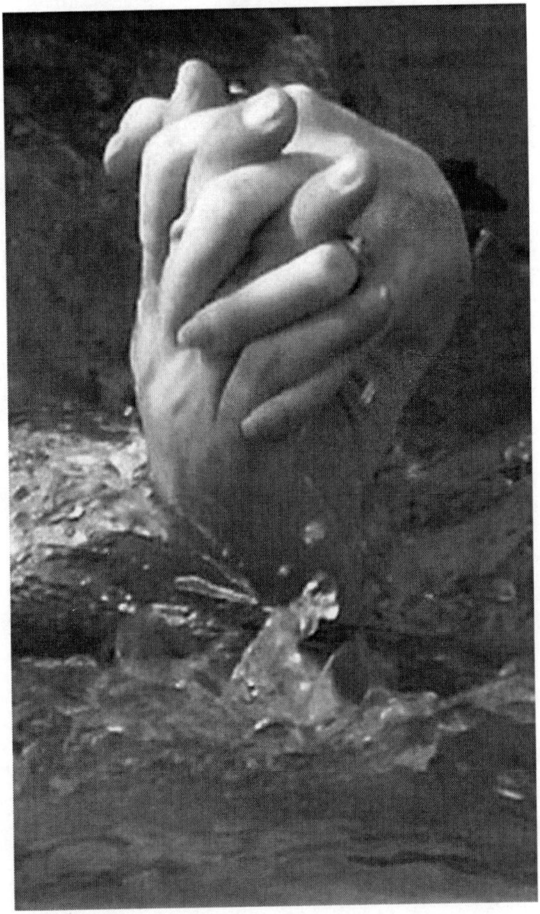

Finding
N-E-D

the story of
Amanda Faye Brown
by husband
Michael W. Brown
told by
Jane MacLean Craig

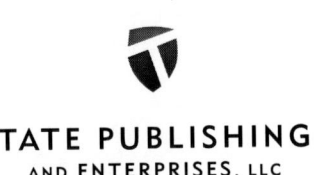

TATE PUBLISHING
AND ENTERPRISES, LLC

Published by Tate Publishing & Enterprises, LLC
127 E. Trade Center Terrace | Mustang, Oklahoma 73064 USA
1.888.361.9473 | www.tatepublishing.com

Tate Publishing is committed to excellence in the publishing industry. The company reflects the philosophy established by the founders, based on Psalm 68:11,
"The Lord gave the word and great was the company of those who published it."

Book design copyright © 2012 by Tate Publishing, LLC. All rights reserved.
Cover design by Shawn Collins
Interior design by Stephanie Woloszyn

Published in the United States of America

ISBN: 978-1-61862-958-6
1. Biography & Autobiography / Medical
2. Biography & Autobiography / Personal Memoirs
12.03.26

To:
My Lord and savior Jesus Christ.
For giving me the strength and courage
to be the husband I needed to be.

Jane MacLean Craig
For taking our story and presenting it
so beautifully for all to see and experience.

The Melanoma Education Foundation,
Nathan Adelson Hospice – Pahrump, NV,
The Pahrump Valley Times,
Mitch Woods and his Rocket 88's,
Ivan Kane's Forty Deuce, Sha Na Na,
Mastertech, Paul and Roberta Kaplan (R.I.P. Paul),
Bob Sachs, Launi Kristopher, Bruce Wallace,
Steve Day, Sherry Phillips Jackman, Dennis West,
Dickie Pride, Josh Groban, Michael Grimm.

And to all those not mentioned
who shared part of our journey...

Thank you all from the bottom of my heart.

—Michael—

Table *of* Contents

Introduction

Tracing the struggle of my wife, Amanda Faye Brown, to survive melanoma, a ruthless and painful variant of cancer, this book is also the story of her relentless bravery in the face of overwhelming odds. Tragically, even today, after billions of dollars have been invested in research, the orthodox medical treatment of advanced melanoma still has limited effectiveness. However, through this book, it is my greatest desire to convey the way in which true love is never dimmed, even when death trumps life. For this reason, I have dedicated myself to fighting this illness, through a medical foundation created in her honor, to battle and bring awareness to this grim and pitiless disease, so that multitudes of others and their families will not be forced to suffer the same cruel fate.

As we chronicle Amanda's tenacious journey, you, the reader, will come to the startling realization that melanoma—a leading cancer killer of young women—has created a battlefield as lethal as any physical combat site. And although I do not pretend to sort out this dilemma in the context of these pages, it is my greatest desire that, at the very least, a universal consciousness will be raised, which will result in more awareness of and dedication to combating this devastating illness.

In this book, I have tried to relay the story through a number of eyes. First, through Amanda's as she moves from childhood, to marriage, to encountering the lethal enemy that would end her young and heroic life; secondly, through my own; and finally, through the memories shared by those family members and friends whose lives she so poignantly touched.

Finding NED is a testament to Amanda's overwhelming courage and unshakeable tenacity in the face of impending disaster to fight this all-too-often preventable disease. It is my most heartfelt wish, that one day some spark—whether philanthropic, research-oriented or creative—will enlarge and perfect our arsenal of tools for taking on this utterly devastating disease.

In Her Own Words

Hello! My name is Amanda, also known to my family and closest friends as Mandy. I was born to my mother, Connie, and father, Dwight, on October 27th, 1974. For the first five years of my life, we lived in Hayward, California.

Just after we had moved to Penn Valley in the northern part of the state, my sister, Kristi, was born. My family had relocated there for a fresh start, and our house was situated on a dirt road in the middle of the country.

After living there a few years, Mom and Dad bought twenty acres of land four miles down the same road. We spent the next six years building a house, tending Mom's garden, and growing up as children, carefree and happy in the country.

With our nearest neighbor miles away, we often ran around naked as jaybirds, building tree forts and playing with all the animals we had at the time…goats, geese, chickens, dogs, and cats.

It was a primitive life, and we actually lived without power or a phone for many years. Finally, Dad got ambitious and hooked up a generator and 12-volt batteries so we could have some power. This was significant because, when the generator was running, we could actually watch color TV.

But though we had this luxury, there were many reminders that our life was essentially a very rural one and that we were progressing one step at a time from rustic warriors on the land to, perhaps, a modified type of country gentry.

For instance, in the beginning we had to set up a fifty-gallon tank on top of the hill behind where we lived so we could siphon water into our home. It took awhile, but we finally got our well up and running.

Yet, although it had its difficult moments, between cutting firewood and clearing and landscaping property, my family kept food on the table for the four of us. Nevertheless, while our carefree life as children was seemingly tied so securely to the world of nature, it came at quite a cost with regard to living in the modern, day-to-day world we were cohabitating. In general, we had to do with hand-me-downs and shopped at thrift stores for our school clothes. But on special occasions like Easter, Mom would make us new outfits that we could call our very own.

Even though we were broke, looking back, I would never trade growing up in the country with the more technically and socially refined lifestyle in the city. In fact, I experienced some of my best (and ironically, worst) moments back on that four-mile dirt road. Still, I believe being raised in that rural environment was good for me, and the lessons I learned there served me well when I moved on to city life. It also enabled me to remember what was truly important and not to get lost in the hustle and bustle of the city and its seductively toxic materialism.

But in our culture, there is always a financial downside if one's skill set is not attuned to a "civilized" environment's survival requirements. My family could make it on the level of man against nature but, in that location, could not prosper in the human marketplace.

Eventually, the everyday struggle put such an increasingly large strain on my family (particularly with regard to my parents' relationship) that they finally separated after seventeen years of trying to make ends meet.

To affect their parting, Mom and Dad sold the house and split up our things, and Kristi and I moved into town to live with my mother. But since she was working two jobs to keep us clothed and fed, we hardly ever saw her. Because my dad couldn't bear to be away from his daughters, he relocated as well, renting a place nearby. Their divorce was finalized sometime shortly thereafter.

A few months later, my mom, seeking greener financial opportunities, decided to move my sister, Kristi, and me to Las Vegas. We arrived in this glittering venue on October 1st, 1989, ironically the date of my parents' anniversary. After eight months or so, my father missed his girls so much that he again followed us to our new hometown.

After several years, my mom decided to remarry. With Dad not living with us and Mom focusing on her new husband and life, I felt a bit out of place in my surroundings. This created somewhat of a rift between Mom and me. Eventually, it was mutually decided that I would move out of the house, even though I was not yet eighteen years old.

Deprived of the family support I had grown up with, life became a bit more challenging for me. I moved in with a couple of female roommates, worked odd jobs, and started to drink too much. I went through a wild stage and had to face some pretty difficult consequences.

These repercussions made me slow down and become more cautious and careful about the way in which I conducted my life. Forced to assume adult responsibilities for the first time, I grew up quickly and came to realize that I was the only one who was going to take care of me. Thus, I decided on a career of sorts and began work as a cocktail waitress, first at Binion's Horseshoe Steakhouse on the famous Las Vegas strip.

Eventually, I had my own apartment, and, although sustaining myself enough to get by, I searched for opportunities to increase my cash flow. Ultimately, I decided to find a job on the newer side of the Vegas strip, with hope of securing a cleaner environment, better money, and nicer patrons.

I soon began waiting tables at the All-Star Café, even though I knew I was not cut out to be a food server. At least, however, I was in the area of the strip where I wanted to work. At the time, I had also sworn off dating men for a while.

But apparently my non-dating vows were not powerful enough to overcome the polite advances of one of their employees, namely, Michael Brown. According to Michael, it took a few weeks for him to work up the courage to talk to me. As soon as he did—and it was a matter of seconds—we became instant friends.

The Woman of My Dreams

Back then I was working the graveyard shift as a bartender at a bar called The Brass Rail. It was off of Nellis Boulevard, a real seedy part of town. It definitely sucked. As I was also living with my mother at the time, I knew I needed a better job to establish my own life, ASAP.

Eventually I found a job potential at the All Star Café, but I needed some training first. So, for a while, I'd work grave at the Rail and then go for training on the south side of the strip when I got off duty. After a short period of time, I found myself gainfully employed as a waiter.

I was working there for about a year when some new employees started to filter in. But there was one who especially caught my eye—a gorgeous redhead with a body to match...ooh la la! She was a new food server named Amanda, and as soon as I saw her, I began to mentally review my recent and very dissatisfying dating history. Sure, I could just jump in and ask her out, but noting her bearing and apparent integrity in all her dealings with customers and management, I wanted to approach her in a very serious way...and at the right time. To me, this was no ordinary woman. If she was, why was I trembling inside?

In all honesty, for the first time in my life, I became a very strategic dating planner. And although I wanted to ask her out right away, I decided she was too important to leave our potential destiny to chance. Hence, I decided to plan my advances in a very careful manner.

As such, I sat back and watched as all the other schmucks asked her out to no avail. Frankly, knowing everyone there at the time, I wasn't a bit surprised at her reaction. Honestly, I didn't think one of them had a chance and sincerely believed I was a much better match for this regal and charismatic beauty.

After about two weeks of seeing her and knowing she had been on a few dates, I could wait no longer and finally started to flirt. As I later revealed to her, my waiting wasn't due to any inherent shyness but rather a carefully laid out plan on my part. I wanted the terrain cleared, with the dead and dying on the battlefield of love clearly eliminated from annoying, day-to-day competition.

Finally the day I planned to make my move arrived, and I cornered her in the back waiter station.

"Hey, Amanda…" I said with all of the enthusiasm and sincerity I could muster.

"I'm sorry. What's your name?" she coolly replied.

"Michael. Michael Brown. What's up?" I queried. "I'm so glad you finally came to visit with me."

Shot down, she casually replied, "No, I thought you were working the grill. I'm waiting for an order."

Regaining my composure, I said, "Actually, I've been wanting to speak with you for some time now." As soon as the words left my mouth, her face suddenly flushed. It was a beautiful color, one that matched her cascading red hair. But more importantly, I knew her reaction was a very good thing, so much so that she forgot to pick up her order. Moving forward, I continued, "Hey, you know, Amanda, I play sax."

Somewhat stunned with grease flying all around us and an order of burger and fries in my hand, she intoned, "Really, you're a musician?"

"That's right," I quickly replied.

Then the inevitable question left her lips. "So why are you working here?"

After explaining that I was seeking nothing more than a steady flow of money, as my gigs were not all that regular, I mentioned that I was playing at the Crown and Anchor that very night and invited her to come and watch me in action. Thankfully, she graciously accepted, as she blushed an even brighter hue. Then and there I realized that my strategy for making this goddess my own seemed to be working, increasing my confidence tenfold. In fact, I felt like a peacock unfurled and ready for action.

Commenting on what a beautiful name Amanda was, she looked at me, sighed, and smiled unforgettably. I knew at that point I was on the highway to heaven! After informing her that I was playing with a group known as Uncle Sugar and the Sweet Daddies (led by my close friend, Timothy Pogue, known professionally as Dickie Pride), she coyly asked which I considered myself to be. At that very moment, my suspicions were confirmed that she most certainly was the *one* for me.

As show time approached, I fortified myself with a few beers. My set hadn't arrived, but neither had Amanda, and I was hoping and praying she'd hurry up. Surfacing with a friend in the nick of time, she sat next to me. Maybe I projected too much, but I had the distinct impression that she and her friend were like Siskel and Ebert waiting for the movie to start. For the life of me, I didn't want to see her vote thumbs-down. In my mind, this had to be my most memorable performance; I needed to kick butt, without question! When it finally came my turn to play, I focused my eyes with laser-like sharpness straight at Amanda, with all the passion in my heart fueling my performance. When a great big smile appeared on her face, I knew I had crossed an incredibly important hurdle on my way to making her my own.

But when I came down from the stage, she gave me a look that I will never forget. I know this might seem very premature in the realm of love and commitment, but I felt her eyes had silently said, "You make me feel differently than I have ever felt before. For the first time, I sense something missing in me has finally come into my life. I feel like you complete me." As I say, the look and its infinite innuendos, though validated by feelings that would soon be articulated, took me by surprise. Perhaps, I thought, my analysis of her reaction was simply an over-interpretation of a pretty young woman's look. Or maybe her smile acted like a mirror to my feelings, which were, although heartfelt, equally premature.

Whatever Amanda's gaze meant, it evoked an incredibly special feeling in me that I had never before experienced. A few moments later, she said she had to go home, and I walked her and her friend to the car. I gave her a hug and said, "I'll call tomorrow." As they drove away, my heart felt like it was skipping! I guess the time for courting had begun. Wow, I thought, my plan was completely on track; and it even felt as though I was ahead of the game!

The very next day, I arranged to come by and take her out to dinner. Secretly, I planned to ignite a really cool fireworks display before our official date began, but I didn't reveal a thing. When I finally took her up to Red Rock and lighted a few off, Amanda was overwhelmed by the gesture. I was pulling out all the stops, if you will, and I could see she was responding in kind.

After the fireworks, we drove to Tropicana and Rainbow. On the way, I stopped at a 7-Eleven. (Yeah, we both smoked at the time.) We went into the store, but when we came out, the car wouldn't start! As much as I tried, it would not turn over. Now I don't know anything about fixing cars. I drive them…that's it. And although I was having a personal esteem self-destruct, Amanda was a good sport about the whole thing. Fortunately, my twin brother lived only five minutes away, so I called him to rescue me from an embarrassing situation; one that I certainly did not want to prolong. Following that debacle, we had dinner, and I held her hand as we walked back to her apartment from my brother's truck, which he had graciously loaned me. As we reached her apartment door, I didn't even try to kiss her. And although it was hard to keep my composure, I knew I had to…the stakes were simply too high for a misstep. As I let go of her hand, she smiled and said, "Good night."

Walking back to the truck, I found myself in a state of utter bliss. Yes, it would have been nice if I had taken her home in a limo, but I was beyond trying to impress. Cupid's arrow had struck a bull's-eye! Every indication of what we had together was showing signs of unwavering solidity. And isn't that what we all want from love? Let's just say that, at that point, whether our choice of transportation was a stretch or a tractor didn't really matter.

The next day I was thrust back into reality when I had to deal with my car's mechanical condition. Although I was slated to contact her, I felt an uneasy wave of embarrassment come over me when I started to initiate the call. Pondering the possibility that I had just blown it with the hottest girl I'd ever known and fearing the ramifications of such, my hesitation didn't last too long, and I sprung back into immediate action.

The fact of the matter was that Amanda was very sympathetic toward the efforts of the previous night. Thank God! Man, did I pour on the charm after that. It was thick, believe me, almost too much, and I wondered if I just might have been pushing too hard.

No matter. I couldn't do other than to keep forging on in my quest for this jewel in the crown known as Amanda. It was my way of spreading those peacock feathers, my general protocol, amped up about a thousand times. I vividly remember one of the first dates I had with her following that night. She had accompanied me to Lake Tahoe for a gig I was playing with Mitch Woods and his Rocket 88's. After going on a short hike, we wound up near the lakeshore. It was a magnificent day as we sat together, just pondering the beauty that surrounded us. I was falling in love, and I knew it! I remember thinking, *Man, am I glad she can see me play with Mitch! I need to impress the heck out of her.* Happily the performance went off without a hitch, with her presence motivating me to give it my all. That night I held her tightly as we watched the town's Fourth of July fireworks light up the entire lake, a mirror of the way I felt in my heart. Amanda looked so damn good…perfect, in a word. Against all cries in favor of slowing down the pace, looking before you leap, being cautious…I was indeed completely hooked.

In retrospect, I think I viewed all women at the time, including Amanda, as python-like creatures, and I was the charmer with the big flute. However, one night, while over at her apartment, she suddenly gave me a strange stare. It was like an emotional cut-off, probably fear induced, propelled by the fact we were moving too quickly in our relationship. Taking my cue, I then decided to lay off the bull crap and get serious. I needed to win her heart and trust, not just to lure her into my romantic little spider web. I needed to risk being myself and knew, innately, that the only way I could win her heart was to risk letting her see the real me, and not the cool, strategic player that had a huge arsenal for nailing women's interest.

Thank the Lord, it worked! After a few more dates, I started to gain her trust and came to realize that she actually liked the real me. In fact, one of the first signs indicating that fact surfaced when, during a visit to her apartment, she confided in me she was about to apply for another job. Naturally, wanting to appear her very best, she began to wash her hair. When I offered to help her out in that regard, she nodded a definitive "Yes," and I followed her into the bathroom. As she began to pull off her top, I tried my hardest to keep a straight face, but inside I was going crazy! Man, what a beauty!

By this time, I could see that she felt safe with me, and I reveled in her newly revealed confidence. She made me feel so special. And although I never lost sight of her tremendous sexual appeal, I quickly came to realize that true love is a feeling that can compare with no other. My heart raced with happiness.

Soon, thereafter, she got a job cocktail waitressing at the Gold Coast Casino. She just went down and applied, and *boom*, she got the job immediately. Obviously, her extraordinarily good looks served as a key, as they always want the most alluring-looking women for such positions.

During the course of my visits to her at work, I noticed the multitude of men who were hitting on her. Although I wasn't particularly fond of this "climate," I found it vicariously flattering at the same time. The truth was, I was proud of having such a hotty for my girl. Of course, there's a downside to being exceptionally good looking, and it manifests itself in that green-eyed monster known as jealousy. Therefore, it wasn't too long before the other waitresses started to make things difficult for her, which ultimately resulted in her being let go.

"I didn't cut it, Michael. I was too slow, too rude, too something," Amanda lamented.

Responding with all of the love and compassion I had in my heart, I asked her, "Are you telling me that you failed in your job?"

"Well," she disappointedly replied, "what else would you call it? They told me I was slow. But, frankly, I'm really fast." Poor darling couldn't see the forest for the trees, and I went on to explain that the simple truth was she was attracting too many customers, with accompanying, very generous tips. The hags merely became envious. This wasn't a matter of performance, but rather the normal reaction of those less "gifted."

She simply looked at me with an innocent strangeness and then shrugged.

By that time, Amanda was living with her sister, Kristi. She wanted to get out on her own, so I paid some bills for her, loaded up a trailer with her things, and moved her in with me on Arville Street, just seven minutes from the strip. It wasn't an optimum situation, but at least we were together.

During our first Christmas season, the apartment complex had a decorating contest, and the first prize was a month's free rent. Spurred by this highly appealing offer, Amanda immediately started festooning the balcony with red and green lights. Her love of the holiday was contagious, fueling our enthusiasm as we adorned the entire area with festivity. Although confident—we were a shoe-in for the blue ribbon—we ultimately were awarded second place. Nevertheless, Amanda was happy, for we knew who the *real* winners were in all that really mattered…*us!*

Simon was my roommate at the time. He was a cook at the All Star Café and a really good guy. Unfortunately, his girlfriend could not be similarly described; in fact, I often thought that peace on the home front could only be found if she had her mouth taped shut. Continuing the white-hot noise emitting from her overly sized mouth throughout the night, Amanda and I had to also endure many hours of her screams of passion, due to our excruciatingly thin walls. There was just no respect shown to her cohabitants of the apartment, and something had to give.

Although Simon's girlfriend made moves to establish her territory (through specific hours, borders, and barriers for us living together laid down), Amanda stood her ground. She was cordial to the lady but very stern at times. She wanted what she wanted and would not let someone else control our space for the sake of a cheap power trip. As far as I was concerned, Amanda was the real one ruling the roost.

Some weeks later, a light rain began to trickle in an open window in our living room. Bearing in mind precipitation in Vegas is such a rare occurrence, Amanda simply couldn't contain her delight. Running out onto the grass below our balcony, she twirled around and around, all the while laughing and giggling like a happy child performing a summer rain dance. As I watched her, I actually felt myself falling more deeply, more irrevocably in love. Realistically, it wasn't too hard to do.

Silence Is Golden

During this time, I was going back and forth a lot to see my dad, Ronnie, who led a highly successful musical trio during the height of the Rat Pack years. A recording artist for Columbia Records, his health had been failing him for some time and, together, we were living the "thirty-six hour days," common to Alzheimer's patients and their caring family members. He was at a home in Corona, California. While this is an expansive story unto itself, I have reserved the telling of it for another time, as this book is exclusively dedicated to chronicling Amanda's courageous journey. Nonetheless, I was extremely grateful for the opportunity to spend time with my dad in the Alzheimer's ward and so thankful that he indicated he remembered me.

Later on, Amanda joined me on a few of those trips. Given everything that subsequently occurred, I cherish the fact that, while we were still dating, my beautiful Amanda had a chance to meet my father. I remember the day she gave him a kiss on the cheek. Chills ran up and down my spine, and I will never forget the feeling I had of speaking to him silently at that moment. "Dad," I said, "this is Amanda, my future wife. She's a doll, isn't she?" And while it's always tough to know what patients suffering from this devastating illness are actually aware of, those like me, who have had to live in its wake, understand there's often a priceless undercurrent of communication between those who know and love each other. Intuitively, I knew that my dad was very proud, for he never could resist a beautiful woman! Although his condition was far from optimal, I know in my heart that if he was still able to talk, he would have said, "Good boy, Michael...she's a beauty!" He said it with his eyes.

One day shortly thereafter, I was with Amanda when we received a call from the hospital saying that my father was not receiving enough oxygen. And although I was some distance away on a job (in Orange County, in fact), my close friend, Keith, as well as Amanda accompanied me as I flew to his bedside. That proved to be one of the greatest gifts of my life, as I did all I could, holding his hand, continually whispering how much I loved him. In something of a trance-like state, I was riveted back to the grim reality of the situation by the stern voice of his doctor who told me that, if he didn't rally soon, they had no choice but to put a breathing tube into him. Knowing my dad as I did, I was keenly aware of the fact that if a breathing tube was inserted, it was the beginning of the final curtain. So I went outside and prayed with Keith on one side of me and Amanda on the other.

It was hard to believe this was happening, and before I went back in, I cried bitterly. It was a good long cry, but I knew I had to get it out of my system before I returned to his side. Miraculously, when I reentered the room, his levels of oxygen intake were improving dramatically. After staying for a few more hours with him, it was clear that he'd dodged the final bullet...at least for the time being. In fact, when we ultimately decided it was safe to leave, his condition had gotten substantially better. "Thank you, Jesus!" I said silently.

Later that night, Amanda commented on how much stronger and clearer my voice sounded. "This is better than Thanksgiving," I shouted, my words resonating with gratitude. Our prayers had been answered, and as such, I had been given the gift of more time with my beloved father.

Over the next few months, as Amanda loyally accompanied me to his bedside visits, I experienced a strange phenomenon, the sense that my father was somehow directly communicating with my girlfriend. Naturally, I knew he couldn't talk, but his love for us both came shining through his weak smile. I'll always have tremendous gratitude for the mercy God showed in allowing my father to get to know my future wife.

Love in Bloom

Early in our relationship, one of our favorite activities was going to the movies. Apparently, it was all my love-addled brain could come up with in terms of recreation. However, any chance I had to hold my wonderful Amanda's hand (especially in the dark) was good enough for me! I guess I was more of a rookie than I thought in terms of designing heavy schedules for dating, but this wasn't what I was used to. My prior experience was two or three hot dates and then good-bye. I had no experience organizing outings when true love was the catalyst for togetherness!

So, one time, after visiting the Orleans Casino with our good friend and neighbor, Daryl, we decided to all go see a film together. After the show, we went out to the parking lot. It must have been twenty degrees or lower, absolutely frigid for our "neck of the woods." Amanda didn't do cold very well, as her body would tense up, and in no time, her chattering teeth would start to sound like a jackhammer. To avoid all that, she started to run to the car in hopes of getting the heater started up quickly. After gaining about fifteen feet on us, her legs stiffened, and, as a result, she fell right on the cold, parking lot asphalt…face first. Witnessing the scene, I ran to her as fast as I could, and when I arrived at her side, she immediately wrapped her arms around my neck, hugging me intensely. I held her up as she started to whimper. Although she undoubtedly wanted to bellow out in pain, she chose instead to be courageous (probably because she didn't want to freak me out anymore than I already was). It was the first hug of many to come that clearly said, "Hold me...I need you right now." At that moment, I felt special to be the man into whose arms she could collapse without fear. I knew with all of my strength I would hold her up and take care of her, and I always did to the very best of my ability. I remember talking with Amanda's mother, Connie, about the future. I told her I wanted to ask Amanda to be my wife, and she reacted with elation, making me very happy indeed. So, with her blessing, I started to plan for the proposal. And I wanted to do it in a very special way.

The propitious moment came when I had a gig at the Derby in Los Angeles with Mitch Woods. Amanda and I had arrived in LA a day early where the show itself was going to last two nights. To save money, we shared a room with Big Daddy Joe Kyle, our stand-up bass player. Connie and Al (her stepfather) wanted very much to witness this momentous event, so the next night they arrived on the scene with some members of Al's family in tow.

As I had alerted Mitch to my plan, we decided to play a song called, "Pink Champagne" (a slow, bluesy-type tune) to lead up to the proposal. It included a big sax solo, during which I would traditionally go around the crowd and play it up with the ladies. But this time I was directing my efforts to just one very special woman in the audience. To add a more intense romantic ambiance to the occasion, I had also arranged for a security guard to hold a bouquet of red roses in the wings. Meanwhile, I nervously checked to see if the family ring Connie had so generously passed down for me to give Amanda was securely in place. Roaming the dance floor, I suddenly stopped (as did the band) when I reached my bride-to-be. Playing with my left hand, I grabbed the roses with my right.

Of course, the patrons on the dance floor didn't have a clue as to what pivotal moment in two young lives was about to unfold before their eyes. I handed my sax to someone to the left of me (I don't even remember who it was, nor did I care at that point). My God...I was about to propose! Suddenly, I dropped to one knee and handed her the flowers. Then, with the ring Connie had given me, I asked Amanda to be my wife. With the screams of the enthusiastic crowd preventing me from hearing Amanda's reply, Mitch, realizing my dilemma, came down with the microphone and put it to Amanda's mouth. And that's when I heard the most beautiful word ever uttered from any human being spoken. "Yes!" Finally I knew that despite all the heartache, searching, and faulty turns in the road, I had found and captured my one true love.

As my fiancée, Amanda continued to display the tremendous character and strength I had come to know and respect in her. To illustrate my point, one day while driving home from Amanda's father's house in Pahrump, a big SUV cut me off. Naturally, I became upset and in retaliation showed him the scar on my middle finger where the lawn mower had almost chopped it off when I was a kid. Okay, okay...admittedly a bit of bad judgment on my part. Anyway, we were at the top of the hill going toward Vegas on Hwy 160 when the driver of the SUV started to pick up speed, barreling toward us from behind. Since there were no turn-offs for at least twenty miles, I reacted by going increasingly faster myself, and, as this guy obviously didn't appreciate my "scar," followed in hot pursuit. With our neighbor, Daryl, in the back seat, Amanda began to scold me. "Did you really have to do that, Michael?"

Naturally, the peanut gallery in the back seat had to chime in, and did so with the words, "That's one ugly middle finger, Mike."

I acknowledged both comments with the reply, "You're right, Amanda, and please shut your trap, Daryl."

As we forged ahead, things became steadily more precarious when I noticed we had hit seventy miles per hour on this seemingly never-ending, long, winding road. Although the tension level in the car was hitting a fever pitch, the other driver just wouldn't let up. Checking the speedometer, I had reached one hundred miles per hour when, finally, I spotted a gas station. Screeching to a drastically slower speed, I hung a left into the station where my nemesis continued in hot pursuit. Following me into the station, he turned on his lights, and as soon as he parked his car, a wave of sheer terror overtook me as I realized that he was a *cop!*

Suddenly, it dawned on me, that although this was also an SUV, it wasn't the same one at whom I had flashed my not-so-subtle obscenity. As the officer approached my window, I felt my stomach doing somersaults, and when he finally arrived, I innocently said to him, "What the heck did you do that for?"

He was not pleased and on the contrary was highly accusatory. "You knew I was a cop," he intoned. "What were you running for?"

With those words, Amanda suddenly went ballistic, saying, "Sir, we had a confrontation with someone who had the same type of vehicle you have. Naturally, we assumed that he was the one following us. It was a mistake, kind of like the one you just made by putting us in jeopardy by forcing us to drive so fast." Well, this only served to incite further anger in the cop, and his expression toughened.

Looking at her sternly, he undoubtedly was about to say something that he could very well live to regret. However, my daring fiancée cut him off at the knees with the comment, "You didn't even put on your lights! How were we supposed to know who you were on that dark road? All we witnessed was someone—we assumed a maniac—chasing us in a big car at one hundred miles per hour."

At that point, I thought I heard him mumble something, but he simply scowled and slunk back to his car. He actually seemed petulant, almost like a kid kicking the dirt because he didn't get his way. Not putting on his lights! Damn, he must have felt stupid. As I drove away, I turned and looked at Amanda and said, "I'm so glad I'm going to marry you!" Basking in her victory, she gave me one of her heart-melting signature smiles. She was so proud of herself, having just slam-dunked that officer. It was great. Daryl, our neighbor, was laughing so hard he hurt his side.

I knew I was in trouble the moment after I gave Amanda her first back rub! I'm pretty darn good at it, if I do say so myself, and she quickly became addicted. In fact, she loved it so much that I had to give her a back rub every single night from that point forward, developing our own personalized system for satisfaction in the process. First, she would have me dig deeply into her torso like I would a man…she could take it. There was a large protrusion in the upper right side of her back, and she would insist that I put my elbow right into it and just press as hard as I could. Of course, we later came to realize that the protrusion was actually an indicator of more trouble on the horizon, but that wasn't apparent at the time. And although the massage hurt her a bit, it also brought her great relief. Whatever she wanted, I tried my best to comply with any and all of her requests. I just wanted her to feel better. In addition, Amanda liked to lie on my back, trying to shape her body to the contour of mine, with the closeness of this position providing me with great pleasure, as well.

I remember a time after one of these special treatments, she returned the favor, and after she was done rubbing my back, she climbed aboard, as usual. Apparently, some air had gotten stuck in-between her belly and the middle of my back, and as she wriggled down more closely, it got squeezed out of the side and sounded like I had just eaten a whole can of Five Alarm Chile! We both started giggling so hard Amanda had to run to the bathroom! I couldn't have cared less as to how seemingly vulgar or trivial the source that ignited the gales of laughter in us was; I just loved enjoying any time at all with her.

Being childless, a huge part of the joy we experienced together arrived in the form of our four-legged "babies," i.e., our exuberant cats. We used to call them "our boys."

The first to arrive on the scene was Sammy, who had a whole set of eccentricities unique to him and him alone. Number two joined the family when Amanda learned that my brother had some kittens that needed homes. I was all for Sammy remaining an "only child," but with one look at the runt of the litter, Amanda fell in love, and Tigger became a Brown. With short, spotted hair, he was given the moniker due to the fact that, like his namesake *Winnie the Pooh* character, the boy could really bounce...and high! I remember the first night he came home with us; so small I could fit him into the palm of my hand. We had just gotten into bed, when Amanda placed the little guy on her chest. Slowly moving his head up to Amanda's chin, Tigger began to purr in an astonishingly resounding voice for such a tiny fellow. Not only did we chuckle at the sheer volume of his purr, we laughed even harder upon catching sight of his adorable overbite. He was just the cutest thing ever. Gazing over at the two of them, I witnessed the birth of a lifelong bond that would serve to provide my wife with immeasurable comfort during the dark days ahead. Tigger simply refused to ever leave her side.

Another afternoon, not long thereafter, Amanda called me from work. She said that she and a coworker were outside when they discovered a little kitty lying in the corner of the backyard, covered with a layer of ugly, red swarming ants. Upon closer examination, they could see that the ants were literally eating him alive, and he was screaming in pain as a result. When Amanda approached him, he summoned up enough energy to jump into her arms, and there he remained (whenever possible) for the rest of her days.

Although he was a male, she named him Mossie (a/k/a Tumbelina), and with good reason. For after she brought him home, Amanda placed the little cat on the bed and started to sing Culture Club's "I'll Tumble for You," something that made him so happy the kitten began to do somersaults! "Boy" number three was now firmly ensconced into our happy little group. In fact, he's still tumbling to this very day every time I break into his favorite song!

Treated like the babies they were and still are, whenever we went to the supermarket, we always got treats for them. (Actually, Amanda and I called them "treaties.") Now Sammy was a freak when it came to those treaties, and being a highly discriminating soul (a trait he demonstrated very early on), only one brand and one brand alone would satisfy his palate… Temptations! Whenever we got back from the grocery store and put our purchases on the counter, Sammy would zero right in on the treats bag. It was very funny to see. Although he tried to open it on his own, much to his chagrin, he never quite succeeded. Hence, he was forced to enact a "back-up plan" to stake his claim, a maneuver which involved him lying down right on the bag and waiting for us to put the groceries away. When that task was completed, Sammy would stand up and start furiously pawing away at sweet Temptations! Inhaling his favorite "vice" like an addict jonesing for a fix, they seemed to disappear with a mere "slight of the paw," very reluctantly sharing what we could quickly salvage for his "brothers" in the process. So naturally, when we wanted the boys to come inside, we would use the treaties bag like a fisherman uses bait. Stepping outside, lure in hand, I'd shout (in my best, deep-throated, Jack Nicholson baritone), "Come on, boys, treaties!" They would soon come galloping toward the house with Sammy, our little "treatiemonger," leading the pack. Amanda never got tired of their homecoming ritual, and every night she would stand on the porch and laugh and laugh when they scurried to her side.

And Then We Were One

Well, the day we had been so anxiously anticipating finally arrived. It was May 6, 2000, our wedding day, a very blessed time for us both. Amanda's years of estrangement from her mother had seemingly melted away and, as such, Connie made most of the decorations and handled a great many other details for the wedding. In fact, we had all become so seemingly close; Amanda and I had graciously agreed to accept their invitation to move into the guesthouse on their property. Not like the apartments we were used to, this was an actual house; and we were both extremely excited at the prospect of setting up our first home there together. When the big day was upon us, Amanda and I both looked like deer in headlights! After all, we were about to be married! As the clock struck four, my brothers and friends lined up on my side, as did Amanda's sister and friends on hers. When the music finally started, my heart raced so fast I thought it was going to jump out of my throat.

I began to hyperventilate, and I remember my brother Rick saying, "Calm down, Mike...Just *breathe!*" However, when the door opened at the top of the stairs, all of my fears were allayed, for there stood the most breathtaking creature I had ever seen. As she turned to walk down the stairs, Amanda looked so beautiful I could barely contain my self. Her aura was nothing short of angelic. *I'm about to marry the most beautiful girl in the world!* I thought to myself. Choosing to walk down the aisle alone, Amanda was stopped halfway by Dwight, her father. "Who gives this woman to this man?" the minister asked.

"I do," replied Dwight. And with those two words, his daughter was ushered into the next phase of her life. Although I remember trying very intently to listen to the pastor, the only words I wanted to hear were, "I do!" And suddenly the moment was upon us. When the pastor asked, "Do you take this man?" her eyes filled with pure love and devotion as Amanda gazed at me tenderly and sweetly answered, "I do!" To say this was one of the happiest seconds I have ever experienced is the greatest of understatements, for with those two words came the dawning of our new life *together.*

My dear friend, Dickie Pride, lead singer of Uncle Sugar and the Sweet Daddies (to whom I previously referred), brought his entire band to play their renowned 'swing' at the reception. So, instead of the traditional, first-dance waltz, my new bride and I did a jumpin' jive dance to the sounds of their incredible beat.

However, despite the elation of the moment, there was a bump on our road to total bliss. For before we left for our honeymoon, a major misunderstanding erupted between Amanda's mother, Al, and us with regard to payment of some of the wedding bills. As a result, it was mutually decided that we would leave their guesthouse as soon as possible. In retrospect, I now realize that Connie and Al were merely trying to help, and I was the one who completely overreacted to the situation, with Amanda simply following my (misguided) lead.

Deciding to put the entire issue out of our minds and deal with the consequences upon our return, we joyfully departed for Rosarito Beach, Mexico, where my big brother from the Big Brothers Organization had arranged for us to use his beachfront condo, to fully embrace our first days together as man and wife. I'm happy to report that as a result, our honeymoon proved to be nothing short of magnificent! Those glorious, love-filled days and the memories we created during them have continued to sustain me during some of my darkest hours. To say the setting was simply gorgeous would be to not do it justice. It was, in a word, Shangri-la! In fact, there is no way to accurately describe the bliss we experienced during that magnificent week—seven days when our future appeared so bright, as they say, "we had to wear shades." With the condo situated right on the beach, we felt as though we were experiencing heaven on earth. Whenever we so desired, we would go out, take a stroll, and check out the shops. And then there was the food. It's honestly hard to explain the sheer scrumptiousness of authentic Mexican cuisine. The lobster was beyond describable, and one of the restaurants even served fried ice cream! We went horseback riding on the beach every morning, and I truly felt I was living a dream. With that said, I'd like to remind readers to completely bask in the happiest moments of your lives, for you never know when the tide will turn.

Two Weeks

As had been decided before our Mexican departure, we had to find a new place to live as soon as we returned. Since I was leaving for Europe soon, my drummer friend, Glen Hill (Stix), offered to let us stay with him. But just two weeks after we got back from our honeymoon (the only fourteen days I had with a healthy wife), Amanda was rear-ended by an older woman while driving home, and as a result, she had to have an interior posterior back operation.

The operation was intense, as they seemed to cut her virtually in half to access the damaged areas. After that, another specialist came in to move her organs over so they could work on her herniated discs. In the process, they had to turn her over and cut her back as well. After the operation, she was in so much pain. I can hardly bear to relive it, but the experience did afford me the opportunity to witness Amanda's signature move: Grace under pressure, the definition of true class. Please bear in mind, this book was not written for my enjoyment but rather to help you get to know the most courageous woman I have ever met. Her reaction to the overwhelmingly harrowing surgery she had endured at that end of the scalpel was just her first demonstration of the "true grit" that would sustain us both to the very end.

Following the operation, I was alarmed at Amanda's appearance. Her abdomen seemed strangely swollen, but according to the nurses, her stomach was distended because it had basically shut down from the trauma in surgery. I vividly remember sleeping in ten-minute increments then waking to press the morphine button for my wife. But when the time came for her to manage her own pain, the protocol was even weirder and more tortuous. Sure, they would give her something to sleep, but tragically, her discomfort was so great that she would awaken shortly after its administration to press her own button in an effort to continuously manage the ultra-intense discomfort.

Upon her release from the hospital, Amanda stayed with Glen's wife, Claudia, while her drummer husband and I went on a Department of Defense Tour of Europe. Back home, Claudia took wonderful care of Amanda, and when I returned, we found a small apartment near Jones and Flamingo (a great location for us) in which to move.

(Dis)Order in the Court

The lawsuit we had initiated after the accident, the cause of her overwhelming injuries, was then about to get underway, and we anxiously waited for the court date to be set. Once it started, our attorney asked the insurance company for the limit ($100,000.00). Of course, we asked five times that amount (small compensation for what Amanda had gone through), but the opposing side always flatly rejected our requests, countering with an absolutely ridiculous amount in return. We were extremely anxious about the impending trial because we needed to have the extensive medical bills Amanda had incurred paid.

Finally the day arrived, and we were ready to get underway. I was not, however, allowed in the courtroom for the proceedings, as I was going to be called to the stand. The first witness our attorney called was the officer that had arrived on the scene, immediately following the collision. Sadly, when it was his turn at bat, he was a no-show. As such, Amanda became unglued, from the acute awareness that there would be nobody else to advocate for our side. At this point, everything hung on Amanda's testimony alone. When she was finally called to the stand, her well-founded anxiety simply overtook her, and she started to cry. Subsequently, when queried about the accident, Amanda reacted very strongly and began to actually weep more violently. The opposition attorneys took advantage of her fragile emotional state by actually laughing at her performance on the stand, suggesting that her breakdown was staged. Obviously, having lived through this hideous time with her, and having had to pilot her morphine infusions through her postoperative state, I knew what terrible nightmares she was reliving through their questioning. Unfortunately, at the end of the day, we not only lost the case but also the "king's ransom" we had invested in the extensive medical intervention necessary to—like Humpty Dumpty—put my wife back together again.

We were later told by our attorney that the jury apparently believed Amanda faked her entire testimony, employing "crocodile tears" to sway them. Of course, nothing could have been further from the truth. It still makes me sick to this very day to remember the unbearable pain she endured as a direct result of that accident and how the attorneys leveraged her unfortunate breakdown to convey to the jury that her so-called "staged performance" was intended to merely score a big payday.

Of course, Amanda was devastated, for she knew, as did I, that we were in serious financial trouble. She cried almost continually for days following the verdict, as she felt she wasn't contributing to our life together, even as I constantly reassured her she already had. To me, this situation only served to reinforce the fact that we both needed to be there for one another, in sickness and in health. Eventually she did see it my way...it's called real marriage.

While still in the process of recuperation, Amanda found a job working at the local university. However, her new employers didn't show much sympathy for her needs. In fact, it would be an understatement to say that the conditions imposed on her in her workplace were formidable. She tried to do a good job and certainly did, but the post simply proved to be too much for her to undertake at the time. Nonetheless, her spelling, typing, and organizational skills were awesome. They were lucky to have her; it's just too bad they didn't realize it.

On the Course

Sometime soon thereafter, we moved into a fabulous apartment overlooking a golf course that Amanda had found for us. Personally, I didn't think she could have discovered a more ideal locale! You see, late every afternoon when the regulars had taken their leave, I hopped the gate ten feet from my door and played a few holes for free! Honestly, I was in seventh heaven.

One day, Sammy somehow got out of our apartment. I had just come home from working all day at the Pala Casino in San Diego when I decided to relax with a few rounds of the sport. As I approached the fourteenth hole, I could hear gales of laughter emitting from our apartment in Amanda's famous jovial tone.

"What happened that's so funny, baby?" I asked. In the background, I could hear someone screaming off in the distance, who turned out to be the guy who hit a ball on the rough, which Sammy scooped up. Apparently, the cat saw the ball, leapt on it, thinking it was a mouse, and put it in his mouth. Without missing a beat, he then took it and ran up to our apartment, dropping it right in the middle of our living room floor. Oh, those crazy kitties! "You think Sammy's a dog in cat's clothing?" I asked.

"Hell, I don't know, Michael, but you better return this guy's ball to him. I don't think I can handle him with a straight face," she said, collapsing again into hysteria. And so I did. I was almost ready to get our little retriever a set of irons, but they didn't seem to make any "cat-friendly" clubs. I guess that besides our boy, there just wasn't any demand!

My sister, Shari, and her family were living in Kona, Hawaii at the time, and we decided to take a trip to visit them. Words can't describe how extraordinary it was! Shari and her husband, Scott, took Amanda and me to a spectacular bed and breakfast, nestled deep in the Hawaiian hillside, which proved to be a little slice of heaven right here on earth.

Just as we got to our room, my wife and I heard a showering noise right below the balcony. Upon closer examination, we found ourselves greeted by the most breathtaking waterfall cascade imaginable. I called Shari to alert her to our discovery, and we all immediately jumped into our bathing suits. After walking down a little hill lined with a glorious array of tropical plants and flowers, we quickly realized that it was also home to some hungry mosquitoes. As I heard my sister scream, "They are biting me"! I laughed so hard I had to sit down! As I gained my composure, we reached the rocky shoreline. Amanda leapt onto my shoulders and began reaching for some bananas that were directly in front of us, ripe for the picking. Because she couldn't quite reach them, she giggled like a little girl, but it was the attempt that mattered.

By then my sister and Scott were already basking in the frigid water. Amanda quickly jumped in with her floaty and shrieked as the cold temperature hit her body. I followed my wife in taking the plunge and, let's just say, I could have sung soprano at that moment! Once we got a little used to the water, we decided to attack the waterfall head on. Amanda and I swam so close to it that all she had to do was lean back to have her hair washed by one of God's many fountains. After our swim, we perched ourselves on a rock that overlooked the whole area and lovingly gazed into each other's eyes as we laughed with pure glee. "Look, baby…just look where we are!" Amanda exclaimed.

As we left what we had dubbed "Amanda's waterfall," she turned to me and said, "If anything should happen to either of us, I want to be sure we put some of our ashes into the waterfall."

I looked at my wife, kissed her sweetly, and replied, "You got it, babe."

But following our return, Amanda's back problems persisted, inciting a long and extremely difficult time of pain. Eventually, her medical team decided she needed to have a micro-decompression operation at the L-5 S-1 vertebra, after which she began leaking a yellowish fluid at the incision site, and although her doctors didn't seem overly concerned, every time she stood up, she got a migraine headache.

Ultimately, after much persistence on our part, she was finally readmitted to the hospital. As it turns out, it wasn't just normal leaking from the surgery site but rather a spinal fluid leak. Unfortunately I had a commitment to go and play with my band in California almost immediately thereafter, but I assured her I'd be back at her side half an hour after my returning flight hit the ground…and I was. However, the moment I entered the room, I was greeted with the sight of

Amanda reaching for the phone, her entire body convulsing. When she saw me, she immediately burst into tears. Apparently she had been convulsing, unattended, for close to an hour. Overwhelmingly concerned about the tube sticking out of her back to drain the fluid, I ran out to get a nurse. When she finally arrived, additional help was immediately summoned. In fact, within three minutes, six nurses were holding Amanda's contorted body down on the bed, while one nurse, apparently in charge, tried to calm her down. She was absolutely terrified and in more pain than I can accurately describe.

The sight of Amanda's body violently contorting, surrounded by a bevy of frantic nurses, thrust me into a mind-numbing state of shock. And although I desperately wanted to help, I could do nothing, as my back was pressed against the wall, both literally and figuratively. With my heart pounding like a drum, I can only describe it as the closest I've ever come to having an —out-of-body experience.

Thankfully, they finally got to the bottom of the problem, which turned out to be caused by the fact that one of her integral drugs had not been dispensed to her. Prior to her release from the hospital, however, we were told by her doctor to get a biopsy done on a suspicious-looking mole on her right shoulder. While it had begun to cause her discomfort when touched, he assured us he was quite certain everything was fine, and it was simply a precautionary measure. Naturally, we immediately booked an appointment with a specialist. And through his ultimate discovery and subsequent disclosure to me, it became the day the music died.

The Long Journey Begins

The afternoon the call came in had started like any other. The sunny skies overhead mirrored the "climate" inside our happy home with the love of my life by my side. Little did we know or could have ever imagined in our wildest dreams (or scariest nightmares) the grey cloud that was about to overtake our lives, irrevocably changing them forever. The biopsy revealed that the "mole" was, indeed, melanoma, and Amanda would require immediate surgery. With my mother next to me, we waited breathlessly for the doctor to reemerge from the operating room. After what seemed like an eternity, he finally did. He told us that, although the melanoma had moved up toward the lymph node in her neck, he was confident in his reassurance that the surgery had arrested any further progression.

As such, we scheduled a follow-up appointment with a dermatologist at a well known skin and cancer center shortly thereafter, and she echoed the surgeon's prognosis that everything looked fine. Although hindsight is always 20/20, Amanda later revealed to me that the doctor, in spite of being well aware of her history, had performed substantially less than a thorough exam; in fact, the specialist had never even touched her. My wife was subsequently scheduled for additional testing at the Imagery and Diagnostic Center of Las Vegas, which we were later to learn was for the purpose of detecting any new tumors. On the way home from the center, Amanda was hungry, and although, if within my power, I would have given her the moon and all the stars if she had asked, my beautiful, red-headed wife merely requested her favorite selection from Jack in the Box.

When the phone rang early that evening, the darkest to date, with many increasingly darker ones to come, it was our family doctor, Dr. Bady. The tone in his voice indicated the news was not good, but little could I have imagined at the time just how horrific the words he was about to deliver truly would be. After hearing him intone, "Michael, sit down, I have some bad news," my entire body went limp and my brain numb. He proceeded to tell me what no loved one ever wants to hear: "The melanoma has spread to Amanda's lungs, and the prognosis is not good." Knowing my wife was just in the next room entertaining some friends, I regained whatever composure I could muster and began the longest walk of my life down the hall toward her. But I never could hide anything from Amanda. With one look at my face, she got up and leapt shakily into my arms. Sensing tragedy was about to unfold, our guests quickly headed for the door, leaving the two of us alone to deal with what no one should ever have to handle.

Dr. Bady recommended we explore treatment options at the John Wayne Cancer Institute in Santa Monica, California, so naturally we made an appointment for their first available opening. Upon our arrival, we were escorted into a room where I found a place to sit in the corner, and Amanda positioned herself on the patient table. After a few minutes, Dr. Piro, Amanda's new oncologist, walked in, accompanied by his nurse. The first thing out of Amanda's mouth was, "Doctor, am I able to have children? Can we freeze some eggs before we start treatment?" Because I was pretty sure what the answer was going to be, I braced myself. As expected, he looked at my wife and, in a solemn tone, answered, "No, Amanda, unfortunately not right now. We need to get you started on treatment right away, and if we take eggs, it will just delay doing what is necessary at the moment." As soon as the doctor and nurse left the room, she began to cry. I stood up and held my wife in my arms. Through her tears, she said, "I'm so sorry I can't give you a baby, Michael." But I simply and directly replied that a child needs his or her mommy, and we had to get her fixed before we could start our family. It was the only way I could think to maintain the hope she was so desperately grasping for.

Man Your Battle Stations...

Although we were in the fight for Amanda's life, there were still good moments during this time early in the "war." With her birthday just days away, my friend, Dennis, and I brainstormed as to how to create the perfect meal, and our solution mirrored my desire to give her everything she wanted, in spades. For instead of just one of her favorite dinners, we decided to prepare them *all!* The menu went like this: fillet mignon, lobster tail, crab, shrimp, and to top it off, country fried steak. Of course, these were accompanied by her favorite sides—potatoes and gravy and all kinds of exotic veggies. In short, a meal fit for a queen...my queen of hearts.

She was so happy that she put her arms around me and said, "I have the best husband in the world!"

I said to her, "You bring out the best in me... because I already have the best wife in the world!" As we sat and enjoyed dinner, Dennis and a fellow musician played dueling pianos, and an utterly glorious evening was had by all.

One night as we slept in our bed—it must have been 3am—we both had a very strange occurrence. We both awoke with unpleasant dreams. Actually it was quite scary.

In Amanda's dream, she was petrified at the sight of black snakes appearing and emerging from her chest. She was screaming, frantically trying to pull and rip these black snakes from out of her chest. But that was not all. At the same time, I had my own dream. (Considering what was about to happen to us, this dream I will never forget.)

I was in a hospital room. There were three or four beds with patients in them. I remember trying to take the place of one of the patients. (I couldn't see that patient's face but I knew I had to try and trade places so they could escape the hospital.) I then pulled the sheets over my head to hide my identity from the patrolling nurse. Then, when the coast was clear, I remember running out of the hospital only to see Amanda waiting there with a bicycle. I jumped up on the handle bars and she started to peddle away. I remember her peddling so fast that I was afraid of falling off. Then I was awakened by Amanda's aforementioned dream.

In Amanda's Words...

The day after celebrating my thirtieth birthday, I had a chest X-ray taken, which revealed a tumor behind my right lung. At my new dermatologist's, a biopsy of skin had also been taken from my left abdominal area. The results came back the same day: I had been diagnosed with Metastatic Malignant Melanoma Stage 4b. They said in January of 2005 that my estimated survival time was somewhere between four to eight months without medication. I've now learned to listen to the doctors but not necessarily believe everything they say. My husband and I are doing everything in our power to prove them wrong. I have agreed to undergo two types of chemo: Taxol and Temodar. We have since been continuing to fight this cancer with everything we have and will continue to do so until I recover.

My third round of biochemo will start on New Year's Eve. I fly out in the morning on Southwest Airlines, arriving in LAX at 10:10 a.m. A friend will pick me up and take me to the John Wayne Cancer Institute to meet my oncologist, Dr. Lawrence Piro. I'll be undergoing another PET scan and CT scan. The following day, December 30th, the scans will be compared to the ones that were taken previously to see if the treatments have had any effect on the melanoma tumors thus far. I am very anxious to receive the third round of biochemo treatments on the 31st of December. My mother will accompany me to the appointments, and then Michael will arrive on January 4th, when she is scheduled to fly back to Oregon. My husband and I will return the following day for a rehydration treatment on the morning of the 5th, before flying back to Vegas together.

However, at the last appointment at JWCI, we got some bad news. Although this first line of defense in conventional therapy was beyond grueling for Amanda, her tumors had actually increased 22 percent in size since starting the treatment in early December of

2004. Clearly, this protocol wasn't working. After she was over the initial shock, Amanda noticed that one of the doctors was smiling. He went on to say, "Amanda, we are changing your course of treatment, as there are some new and exciting options for you now." But their explanation of the specifics was very confusing. Fortunately, Connie subsequently did many hours of research on the Internet and was able to explain it to us a little better.

Apparently, by law, the doctors have to try chemotherapy on a cancer patient first because it is FDA approved. Of course, we all know that chemo has been around for the last twenty or so years with unreliable results. The truth is, many patients die while being treated with this less than state-of-the-art therapy. In fact, it is actually considered a "success" if the tumors do not grow more than 20 percent larger during chemo treatment, and the doctors are not allowed to try anything else during its course. I don't know who made this scale up, but in my mind, if the tumors are getting bigger, it is *not* doing its job. Period. Regardless, from their perspective, only when the tumors have increased by more than this percentage is the therapy considered a failure.

Once that occurs, however, the door is opened to many more choices, such as "experimental" medications, which are not yet FDA approved. So, to us, it was something of a blessing in disguise that Amanda's tumors had passed their "benchmark," and she "reaped" the first part of the benefit by not having to endure another grueling round of biochemotherapy. Instead, after just one more test, I was able to take her home.

The alternative treatment the doctors wanted to try was MDX 10-20. For that to be effective, she, like approximately 40 percent of the Caucasian race, had to have the HLA-A2 protein in her DNA. She took the blood test before leaving, and we all prayed for a positive result. If Amanda proved to be HLA-A2 negative, the doctor's second choice of treatment was another jumble of letters and numbers known as ABI 007. As both of these drugs were highly recommended, we were assured that, whatever the outcome, she would be starting on the latest medicinal weaponry as of the third week of January 2005. In the meantime, she was working out to sweat the chemo toxins from her body and staying on a strict diet. Very importantly, she had to avoid any herbs or vitamins that would alter her liver enzymes. Otherwise, she would be disqualified for the trials.

In Amanda's Words...

Unfortunately, I haven't been able to receive either of the suggested medications yet. They found two additional brain tumors and will have to radiate again. 007 ABRAXANE— a.k.a. "'Taxol in a Bubble"—is the next treatment I'll be trying.

The sessions were going to take the whole week, as she had to undergo biochemo (a combination of Interferon and Interleuken) again, per the rules set forth by the insurance company. I imagined it as kind of like jumping through hoops until you hit on something that proved effective. The amount of courage she was displaying was utterly blowing my mind. The day we were scheduled to go to the hospital, I'll never forget Amanda calmly saying, "Well, let's do it!" She was just unbelievable. When we got to her room, I staked out a little area where I could lay down, as I knew this was going to be a grueling time for both of us.

The first nurse who came in to see her was a girl who was clearly upset about something (boyfriend, job, family…who knows). All I remember was her treating us like we put starch in her underwear. The next in line was the night nurse, a young Asian man. And I have to say, he was the most gentle and kind soul I could ever have hoped for. Genuinely concerned and helpful, he even made Amanda laugh in the face of tubes and wires running everywhere. He was a prince in my eyes.

The drugs pumped into her body that night started to take effect immediately. Her skin turned a very bright red, and sweat poured out of her like a trickling faucet. There's no other way to describe it; the treatment was nothing short of *barbaric*. I slept that whole time with one eye open. As it turned out, it was a very good thing because, unfortunately, she could not hold her bladder or bowels. With the chemo in control of her body, Amanda would also vomit uncontrollably. Although she tried to get out of bed silently so as to not wake me, I would get up anyway and help her to the bathroom, which, although only six feet away, seemed at the time like a mile. After she was able to relieve herself, I'd help her back to bed.

She had two or three doses of chemo a day...everyday for a week. Then, the test results we had been breathlessly awaiting came back: Not good. But instead of crumbling to the floor, like I was about to do, she lifted me up and said, "I know I can do this. I'm tougher than melanoma." This was one of our first hospital battles and, unfortunately, far from our last. But I knew if there was a chance, I was with the girl who could win.

Forging On

Amanda tended to be very uneasy about the way I handled a car on the road, and the fact that I had been an amateur racecar driver for a number of years only served to exasperate her fear. Undoubtedly insecure due to the aforementioned accident, she would continually remind me to stop moving so fast. "Slow down! Let them get the ticket," my wife would roar. And she was right, of course. I remember one time, Amanda had a doctor's appointment in Los Angeles, but because I had to work the night before, we couldn't leave until 5:30 a.m. She was going to drive the first leg of the trip to Victorville while I slept, and then I was going to take the wheel. Awakening with my head on her lap, I rose up to see where we were. Next stop: Montclair, California! I looked at her and said, "Baby, you're about one and a half hours too long in the driver's seat. You didn't have to do that, honey." She just smiled, happy in the knowledge that I had gotten some much needed rest. That was so like Amanda, letting me sleep when she was the sick one.

In Amanda's Words...

Michael and I spoke with the doctor and found out that I do not have a certain protein in my DNA needed to try the first treatment, MDX 10-20. Instead, I'll be trying the second one they mentioned, ABI-007. I'll be going to the John Wayne Cancer Institute on January 19th for a CAT scan to see if any of the tumors have increased in size and also to have an MRI of the brain performed to rule out any new metastases to that area.

As of today, the doctor says that my survival rate lies between four to six months without the intervention of any medicine. This is such a short amount of time, and needless to say, I am in quite a lot of shock. I pray that the doctors are wrong. I sincerely hope they are. Thankfully, I will be starting the medication, ABI-007, on January 20th, a week earlier than originally scheduled, as we have no time to waste. As such, we will be making a weekly trip to JWCI for treatment, every Thursday for three weeks, and then off for one week. This will have to be continued until a cure is found.

The most recent update from my last visit to JWCI is very distressing. Michael had accompanied me to get my scans done, and the following day we got the results. Although the good news was that none of the tumors "inside" my body had grown since stopping the biochemo treatment, we were also informed that the tumors residing in fatty tissue—the ones I can feel—have grown slightly. In addition, they found two more small two- to three-millimeter tumors in my brain, one on each side of the frontal lobe. These findings changed the method of their attack immediately. I now need a stat Gamma Knife Procedure at USC to radiate the tumors, and I am no longer eligible for the free trial medication ABI-007 because of the new brain findings. Dr. Piro suggested several other forms of chemotherapy (commonly reserved for malignancies in the ovaries, breasts, and non-small cell, lung cancers) to be used in conjunction with my current treatment. Please keep us both in your daily thoughts and prayers.

The Gamma Knife

The Gamma Knife allows the neurosurgeon to perform an act of virtually bloodless surgery due to the fact that no actual incision is necessary. Thus, the Gamma Knife can function as an alternative treatment for removing benign and cancerous lesions of the brain, which are characterized by sudden bursts (paroxysms) of face pain. It delivers, in one treatment, a single, high dose of ionizing radiation with as much as 201 beams of gamma radiation directed at the lesion with immense precision. The goal is to spur the lesions to slowly decrease and dissolve. It is currently considered, by virtue of various clinical studies, a good choice for small to medium, clearly delineated tumors or malformations and may be used singularly, in conjunction with radiotherapy or in addition to more conventional surgical procedures. In order to operate, local anesthesia and mild sedation is customarily applied along with a head frame to restrict movement while conducting the procedure. This requires delicate and precise, computer-directed measurements. The treatment itself can take an average of a half an hour to a full hour, with follow-up after the operation every three to six months.

I remember waiting in the room with Amanda before the nurse came in and escorted her away for the Gamma Knife procedure. I took a walk and impulsively called one of the dancers at the Forty Deuce (where I was currently playing). While we talked, my heart was breaking, my mind screaming for someone—anyone—to help us. Fortunately, my friend Erin (who truly loved Amanda) was on the other end of the line, just listening and letting me vent.

What a good friend! I thought when I got off the phone with her. As I walked back into the room, the nurse said my wife was done and that everything went well. I almost started to cry right then and there but held back the tears for the benefit of my dear Amanda, who at that point was sitting up in bed. I immediately went over and held her ever so gently as I kissed her. She looked at me while stroking my cheek with her hand and murmured, "I'm okay, baby. I'm okay. I love you."

How can she be so strong, given what just happened to her? I asked myself. But then it hit me: She not only had the love of God in her heart but my undying devotion as well. What more could a girl want? Naturally, I was joking, but there was a deeply spiritual element of truth to it, as well. The bottom line was that she was at peace.

Soon thereafter, we were told that the option was there for Amanda's spot to be held in the ABI-007 trial, but we'd have to wait another month without any additional medication or treatment. Although the drug was slated to go on the market for breast cancer within the next several weeks, as previously mentioned, it would have been extremely expensive to buy it, whereas the trial medication would have been free.

We waited at USC for a good two to three hours, hoping to be fit in the same day we received the news that Amanda needed more surgery. But the nurse came back and said that the soonest time would be the following morning, so we agreed to return then and went on our way.

In Amanda's Words…

Now we also needed to get lodging again and change the plane reservations and car rental. Michael would have to take another night off work, as well as miss a photo shoot for Player Magazine. Of course, I was the only one worried about that. Michael was not concerned at all. He just remained, lovingly, by my side.

I am thankful that my husband is such a world traveler. He has responded wonderfully and has taken care of every detail with a few phone calls. Not much stress for me. Thankfully, the Forty Deuce was able to find a sub to fill in for him that night.

Once all of this was accomplished, we decided to get some dinner near where we had stayed the night before. After receiving an overload of information that day—changing plans for the course of treatment and coming to grips with the fact that I was going to undergo another brain radiation surgery the next morning—I slept mostly all the way through the night. We awoke just in time for Michael to drive me back to USC for the procedure. I went in, and they accessed my Port-a-Cath.

A strange little device was placed in the upper chest area under Amanda's skin that contained a small reservoir connected to a major vein. The Port-a-Cath device helped to administer chemo into her venous system, the purpose of which was to prevent leakage of the poisonous chemo from a vein into nearby tissues. And while this is more likely to happen if the vein is in the arm, there were so many injections to that area, there was a risk of running out of veins.

Anyway, it all went pretty well, probably because Amanda knew more of what to expect. Also, they gave her some relaxant this time when the radiation was administered, as she was very claustrophobic in the tube during the prior treatment. But just before we were ready to leave, they informed us that after they had performed radiation on those two mets, their MRI had picked up two more! Shock! Now a total of five brain tumors! Apparently, their MRI scans slices two millimeters thick with no gap. The other regular MRI scans at five millimeters thick with a one-millimeter gap in between slices. Needless to say, now that we had this information, we were trying to insure that her future scans would be performed with USC's MRI machine or one similar to it.

In Amanda's Words...

On January 25, we're scheduled to drive to Santa Monica to get medicine from Dr. Piro and then turn straight around and drive back home to Pahrump, NV. My doctor said he didn't want to waste any time getting me on medication. I also have an appointment on February 1 to go back to USC for the third Gamma Knife procedure. As soon as we know more, I will update.

We love you all, God Bless!

The last Gamma Knife procedure, her third, was much more uncomfortable than the first two. They radiated the two tumors that we already knew about, but unfortunately, they found another small one that must have come up in the ten days since the last procedure. Luckily, they were able to radiate that one at the same time. To get to the sixth one, they had to maneuver the metal holder around Amanda's head and screw it in through her left temple muscle.

This procedure was extremely painful for her, and the area was sore for days following. It affected her jaw to the point that she was barely able to open her mouth, even to eat, yawn, or talk, and as such, she was forced to *drink* her veggies until the area healed more. She also had to add extra bandages for the first few days because her temple area was weeping and very swollen. However, once she was able to open it to the air, healing progressed. Still, her head remained very painful in the eight places they had to screw in the metal contraption, and her hair was also starting to thin from the medications, eventually coming out in strips.

In Amanda's Words...

Michael and I drove down to Santa Monica on the 8th of February, where I received my second infusion of Taxol. This time, they gained access to my Port-a-Cath without much discomfort. We stayed for two hours, just long enough for the infusion, and then headed right back home. That night, I had the first dose of my new medicine, Temodar. Unfortunately, one of the major side effects of the medication is neuropathy in the feet and hands as well as nausea and/or vomiting. I've found that my feet are most always throbbing and fairly sore since being on this medicine. Luckily, my hands don't throb. They only spasm from the previous neck injury I incurred during the car accident in 2000. My feet, however, wake me up in the middle of the night on occasion. But, I'll keep up with it because it's proving effective for a family friend of ours, Cass, whose brain tumor has shrunk while on Temodar.

Fortunately, we were able to work it out so that Amanda could have her infusions in Pahrump starting the following Tuesday, a small blessing that made things substantially easier on us. But a few days before receiving her latest treatment, my wife ran out of the sample pack of Kytril they had given her for nausea. Although she tried taking a regular anti-nausea pill, she still got very sick from the Temodar. The first morning, she woke up with her mouth watering, followed by the instant need to vomit. After throwing up three times in rapid succession the next a.m., she'd had enough, and she got a prescription for Kytril from her primary care physician. However, when the pharmacy called, they informed us that even with our insurance, it would cost $2,400 for a month's supply! Naturally, we couldn't afford this outrageous price, which was heartbreaking because it worked so well on her nausea. I then asked the pharmacist if they had a similar chemotherapy anti-nausea medication. And although they did, it was only $300 cheaper. Dr. Piro called in an alternative prescription with a copay of just five dollars (more in line with our rapidly dwindling reserves). We just prayed it would work. The oncologist also sent her a few more samples of the Kytril—enough, at least, for a few more days.

In Amanda's Words...

I enjoyed a fabulous Valentine's Day with Michael. We invited my sister, Kristi, and her boyfriend, Craig, to join us for dinner and enjoyed a wonderful meal on the outside patio at the Border Grill at Mandalay Bay Hotel & Casino in Las Vegas. Kristi made us a really good sugar cookie, and I splurged and ate sugar (forbidden "fruit," as it feeds cancerous tumors). But, hey, it was Valentine's Day!

After dinner, we went to where Michael works, Ivan Kane's Forty Deuce Club, for a private party held by Maxim Magazine. They passed around chocolate-dipped strawberries, which were imported from Australia. I ate about five of them, and they were jumbo size! It was a good dessert to accompany the halibut that I had for dinner. As always, I was so proud of my husband's performance. He did an extraordinary job!

Following the show, we drove back to our friend Dennis's house and slept there for four hours until 6:00 a.m., when we headed out to beat that well-known path back to Santa Monica. I slept most of the way down and back this time. We arrived at John Wayne Cancer Institute just in time for my appointment at 11:00 a.m.

I had my third infusion of Taxol accompanied with Benadryl. Michael caught a little sleep while I was getting my transfusion. I felt so bad for him, my poor, sleep-deprived hubby. He had to work again that same night! After we finished, we ordered some food to go from IHOP, got in the Pontiac, and drove back to Vegas. We returned in time for Michael to catch an hour of sleep at Dennis's before working another scheduled party at the Forty Deuce. I stayed with Dennis in Vegas until Michael got back from work around 2:00 a.m. He had gotten his fourth wind by then and drove us home (me in my pajamas) to Pahrump. As soon as we got home, I took that night's Temodar, and we fell asleep.

The next week Amanda wound up getting some kind of bug—a head and chest cold with a very sore throat. She called Dr. Piro, who phoned in a prescription for the antibiotic, Cipro, which seemed to ease her symptoms. After a couple of days, although still not feeling 100 percent, she was nonetheless able to be up and around. Luckily, I had just taken the first few days off from work I'd had in more than a year…four days of freedom from that "grind." The timing couldn't have been better, either, as my poor wife really needed my help.

In Amanda's Words…

Of course, Michael was more than happy to take care of me, fluff my pillows, draw me a hot bubble bath, make me some tea, and later give me a nice massage before bed. Yes, I do have a wonderful husband who I absolutely adore. I am definitely blessed in love!

We confirmed Amanda's appointment for the Taxol Infusion for the following Wednesday with Dr. Kat at the Las Vegas Cancer Center in our hometown of Pahrump—a huge relief for us both. Her primary care physician, Dr. Bady, who had become a good friend, called some people and got it lined up for us. He's a really decent man. Best of all, this was the first week that we didn't have to drive five hours or fly an hour to go down to Santa Monica. So naturally, there was much less stress all around as well as significantly lower expense.

Since she had just run out of the samples of Kytril the night before, Amanda decided to try Compazine for nausea because the price for Kytril (as previously mentioned) was simply too prohibitive. We hoped and prayed it would take care of the inevitable vomiting that would follow her treatment. Amanda had also recently read a couple of books that stated parasites were prevalent in cancer patients. She therefore decided to get tested for them when she got her blood checked for the white blood count. The blood count test was to see what state her immune system was in. Battling that head cold along with cancer really served to only reinforce the importance of maintaining as healthy an immune system as possible.

In Amanda's Words...

It is now the last week of February, and I have been feeling better since recovering from that bug last week. I'm almost done with the antibiotics.

After running out of the samples of Kytril, I have been taking Compazine for the nausea that comes along with the Temodar. The Compazine had been working all right until this morning, but because I am supposed to take the anti-nausea pill an hour before taking my eight pills (130 mg) of Temodar (and as I didn't get back from my dad's house until late last night), I took the Compazine too soon. As such, I awoke this morning at 7:00 a.m. and got sick. I'm now guessing that the trick is to make sure to take the anti-nausea pill at least an hour before taking the Temodar. Another bit of good news: Cathy, a nurse at JWCI, is sending me more samples of Kytril.

I was trying to do my yoga the other night and found it harder than usual to balance on my feet. Since I started taking Taxol, I've experienced neuropathy, which seems to get worse with each infusion. However, it looks like the Taxol is working because a tumor on my left cheek has noticeably decreased in size! My oncologist in Vegas, Dr. Michaels, said that if the neuropathy gets worse, he will reduce my dose.

Although Amanda was supposed to get her Taxol infusion done in Pahrump later that week, they neglected to tell her that they were short a chemo nurse and wouldn't be doing infusions there for another few weeks. Therefore, I got her an appointment in Vegas at Comprehensive Cancer Center with Dr. Michaels the next day, and she had the infusion done then. They did more blood tests, which revealed she was also now anemic. Her WBC (white blood count) had gone up from a few days prior, but her RBC (red blood count) was down. So to help that, they gave her another drug with the infusion, along with Benadryl, which always knocked her out cold. She slept halfway through the treatment, the hour home from Vegas to Pahrump, and into the night, finally waking at around 10:30 p.m.

Taxol and Temadar were the chemo treatments that she started. Taxol is a product that comes from tree bark, and Temadar is prescribed for people that have brain mets. It is one of the only chemos that will break the blood-brain barrier.

I could see past the courageous front she was putting on for me. I saw her real emotions: Unbelievable *terror!* I kept telling her how strong she was and that this was almost over. "Just a little more, honey, and you'll be done!" Amanda got right back in the ring and started fighting another round. Come to think of it, she never got out of the ring. She fought every single minute of her life.

Dancing on Her Nerves

In Amanda's Words...

I had a Taxol infusion yesterday. They lowered the dose by fifty percent this week to see if the neuropathy would get better.

Michael took Kristi, Dennis, and me out to the Border Grill the other night, and although the dinner and company were wonderful, I noticed neuropathy-type feelings in my right pinkie and ring fingers. Later that night, as I was answering e-mails on the computer, the same feeling swarmed over my right shoulder, arm, and hand. It got so bad I wasn't able to type with my right hand. You all know how much I enjoy typing, and although I haven't had my whole shoulder feel that way since then, my right hand continues to give me trouble.

My hair is really starting to thin out now from the treatments. I can finally empathize with middle-aged, balding men! The other night my scalp hurt terribly. I tried lying on an ice pack, but even the weight of that against my hair follicles was painful. It feels similar to the neuropathy in my feet—a pins-and-needles kind of sensation.

In an effort to boost her immune system, Amanda began a diligent search for alternative treatments to accompany the chemo, looking high and low for someone who could provide such additional support.

In Amanda's Words...

Last Saturday was a sad day. A dear friend of ours, Glen "Sticks" Hill, tragically passed away. Thankfully, he was home with his wife (who had so tenderly cared for me) when his heart stopped. He had been on chemotherapy for seven months with squamous cell cancer and other difficulties. Michael and I had just visited him in the hospital. I will never forget my good friend, Glen. He will be missed by so many.

Trying to de-germ our entire house is a big chore, but one we're accomplishing as time permits. Hopefully, while off chemo for these two weeks, I will be able to get my immune system back up again. Then, I'm planning on taking on another round...until this cancer is gone.

Although bright spots in her desperate fight against this devastating disease were few and far between, we did receive some encouraging news in conjunction with the results of the PET and CT scans. All of the tumors throughout Amanda's body were "stable," meaning they hadn't changed in size and those in both of her lungs had even gotten smaller! In addition, there were no new metastases in her brain, and the ones they radiated were shrinking, with one disappearing all together! Upon hearing this, my wife literally leapt with joy into my arms, as we simultaneously laughed and cried together. And although the doctors couldn't pinpoint the specific reason for this seeming miracle, Amanda was absolutely adamant about sticking with her routine of Taxol/Temodar, juicing, Xango, and yoga. Hey, whatever was working, we just hoped and prayed it would continue to do so. I vividly remember her gazing into my eyes at that moment and saying, "I'm going to beat this, Michael! I promise!" Giving up was never part of my incredibly stoic angel's agenda.

In Amanda's Words...

We drove to Vegas today to meet with Dr. Michael and start my second round of Taxol treatments. He noted that I had above average reduction of tumor size throughout my body, not just in the lungs! He also said that after three or four more sessions, I might be near NED (No Evidence of Disease).

We've got this cancer in our sights now; this is no time to let up. Nutrition-wise, I am continuing to juice even more than previously, in addition to taking certain herbs. I am putting Xango in my fruit shakes, too. It makes them taste sweeter, and I can almost feel how much healthier they are for me. I have also cut out red meats, pork, and most shellfish because of their high animal fat content. Trying to "starve my tumors," you could say. And of course, God is the reason for all my recent good fortune. He watches over and touches my life.

The "Hits" Just Keep on Coming

S adly this reprieve was very short lived, as Amanda's WBC (white blood cell count) was then so low they couldn't do the chemo treatment. Her feet and hands hurt so badly that at times she would just cry out in pain and frustration. I tried mightily to provide her with some relief by rubbing her feet and fingers; however, as the neuropathy progressed, she couldn't even tolerate that. It was simply too painful for her to be touched.

In Amanda's Words...

Our five-year anniversary is tomorrow, and Michael has reserved a room at the Mandalay Bay for Friday and Saturday night. Whatever we do, it will be a wonderful experience for me spending quality time with the love of my life, "Downtown" Michael Brown.

Our anniversary was very special. A friend helped me get a beautiful suite with a high-rise view, and Amanda loved it. I got her to take a Jacuzzi to try and relax, and although it did seem to help a bit, I could still see the pain on her face. She just wasn't feeling well. All the chemo and running around and stress and well...you know. But the bed was very soft and comfortable, and I was so relieved when Amanda was able to lie down and not scream out because of the pressure of the sheets. Yes…just the slightest touch would hurt. I mean, even the wind blowing on her sometimes caused pain.

In Amanda's Words…

This past Tuesday we went to the oncologist, and thankfully, Dr. Michael's nurse, Judy, was able to take my blood via the Port-A-Cath. She also gave me the Nulastin shot I needed to get my white blood count back up. I now seem to have "chemo-brain," which Judy said is a normal side effect of this treatment. It affects my short-term memory the most. Sometimes, I'm in mid-conversation and forget what I'm talking about. The only way I know to describe it is that it's like a brain cloud that comes in and fogs up all my thoughts.

The following week we drove to Santa Monica where Amanda received PET and MRI scans and, as the results were going to be ready the next morning, we stayed the night and returned to Dr. Piro's office early in the a.m. to see what they revealed. It turned out to be a *great* day when we learned that all of her tumors were currently stable with no new ones in sight!

While, naturally, my complete focus was on my wife's health, the situation was taking a toll on me as well. For in addition to all that was involved in her fight for life, I was playing with Sha Na Na at the Suncoast Casino Showroom during the evening and then back at the Forty Deuce to do the same throughout the late night. As such, I became very run down and caught a terrible cold. Fortunately, Amanda's dad was able to accompany her to her chemo treatment so I could rest during the day.

In Amanda's Words...

Thankfully, Michael got rid of his cold. Unfortunately, he gave it to me. The first day I had a sore throat, the second ushered in total head and sinus congestion, and the third brought a dry cough. And then it went into my lungs. Even so, my white blood cell count was high enough on Tuesday for me to receive an 80 percent dose of chemo. My red blood cell count is still low, but we are hoping it will go up in time. I started back on my third cycle of Temodar tonight and, having been off of all chemo for a while, I am really starting to feel better.

I had high anxiety just knowing I had to start chemo treatments again. I've noticed a huge difference in how my body feels off chemo as opposed to how it does when I'm on it…like night and day. Oh, I am also easily agitated and just in an overall bad, depressed mood. Yes, the chemotherapy is holding the cancer at bay, but I feel like it's also taking a very valuable piece of me with it. My body is trying to fight off this cancer, while at the same time trying to recover from the toxicity of the chemotherapy.

We decided to put on a benefit at the Forty Deuce Club to raise money for Amanda's medical expenses. I thanked God we have some really good friends that showed us such care and compassion at a time when we couldn't have needed it more.

The Winds of Change

A t this point, Amanda was giving serious consideration to stopping the chemo after four months of horrible side effects. However, when she shared her thoughts on the matter with our families, friends, and doctors, their reactions were universally unsupportive, stemming from overwhelming concern, but she was convinced that the cancer could be cured through nutritional therapy.

Initially, she decided to try and compromise by doing the chemo in conjunction with the nutritional approach, but she was told she'd have to be off the chemotherapy, completely, for the nutritional therapy to be effective. She had been saving all she could scrape together to go to the Whole Life Learning Center in Big Bear, California, and we were so grateful that the benefit would help to defray some of the cost. Constantly researching everything she could possibly find on the subject, she came to really believe that she could cure her cancer through diet and enzymes. It had, in fact, worked for some other stage IV melanoma survivors with whom she spoke; a few had even been cancer free for over twenty years. She rationalized that if it had worked for them, then why not her?

Amanda firmly believed that she wouldn't be able to tolerate the chemo much longer. So not even halfway through the latest round, she decided that she'd had enough. Her body was completely rebelling, and so with steely determination, she set out to find an alternate route to treating the illness, employing a wholesome, nutritional approach.

She decided to retreat to her mom's home in Oregon for a week to just relax and think carefully about her options in the beautiful nature that surrounded it.

In Amanda's Words...

Visiting my mother in Mill City, Oregon the past week was just the medicine I needed. It was absolutely beautiful, and I remember how thick the air was with oxygen and how good it smelled. I could see green for miles and miles.

I've been off the chemo for a week and a half now, and am starting to feel so much better. However, since the results while on it have been promising so far, I reluctantly agreed to finish out this first set of treatments. I should be done with them sometime around September of 2005. After that, the doctors say, I *have* to go off the chemo for a few months. At that time, I plan to spend two weeks in the Wellness Center in Big Bear on the Gerson program. They say that for it to work to its full potential, the patient should continue the therapy for two years. After following it for a few months while off chemo, I will, of course, get scanned to find out how Gerson is working for me.

Yahoo! My hair is growing back! It's about an inch long and starting to fill in nicely. Mom spotted four gray hairs on my head. I wonder why! It seems to be growing in a medium brown with possible red highlights. I am still having the neuropathy pretty badly in my feet.

My coworkers and musical friends threw the benefit at Ivan Kane's Forty Deuce Club in Mandalay Bay during the week Amanda was away in Oregon. We collected enough to pay for her medical insurance way in advance as well as for two weeks treatment at the Wellness Center that Amanda had been so looking forward to attending. She had just such high hopes that this was going to be the defense that would position her on the winning side of her monumental battle.

My wife was becoming very worried and confused about which course of treatment to follow; there were so many possibilities and just as many conflicting opinions. And by then, we were getting almost nothing but bad news. Sometimes, Amanda and I would say a prayer. I would open up the Bible anywhere and just start reading. More often than not, it was something pertaining to what we were going through. It always gave Amanda comfort knowing God was continually with her.

In Amanda's Words…

As I mentioned before, while in Oregon, I decided to finish out this round of chemo before I start Gerson 100 percent. After returning home though, I began to think about stopping the treatment sooner rather than later. I'm feeling so much better, and I believe I have found a way to get healthy again through nutritional therapies. Michael and I are going to Calvary Chapel tonight. I will continue to pray about this decision and I will wait to receive more guidance before making any drastic changes.

I went to a certified nutritionist in Vegas yesterday and talked with her about the Gerson program. She had never heard anything about it. I expected this since she is in mainstream medicine. I asked her to look at what the Gerson therapy calls for and see if it would cover all my nutritional requirements. After doing all the calculations, she told me the diet did, indeed, support them. It showed remarkably high numbers for beneficial vitamins and minerals, which must be why so many cancer patients have had such good results. This therapy seems to give the body what it needs to rebuild and feel good, while leaving out the things that feed and shield the cancer cells from the immune system.

The only thing she was concerned about was the protein intake under the program. It's only 43 percent of what the recommended daily allotment is. This does not alarm me, though, because in the course of my research, I've discovered that there is a strong correlation between overconsumption of animal products and all diseases. To help cure cancer, one must cut down the protein and fats in their diet.

In the initial phase of Gerson (while cleansing the body of cancer), you are supposed to cut out all animal products. After a few years on the regimen, and once the cancer is gone, some animal products are allowed back in moderate amounts. Did you know that the outer covering of a malignant tumor is made up of a fibrin protein? This protein hides the tumor and acts as a shield from the immune system.

According to Amanda's July 11th scans, everything in her brain and body was still stable. One of the lymph nodes seemed to have gotten bigger, but Dr. Piro said, "That is to be expected." We were thankful there were no new lesions and that the tumors were stable but extremely disappointed that no reduction in their size was apparent.

Dr. Piro thought it best that she remain on both chemotherapies for the time being, and while Dr. Michaels agreed with her sticking with the Temodar, he was advocating a switch from Taxol to Thalidomide due to its less toxic effect on the body (although it did have a higher risk of producing blood clots). We waited for her doctors to agree on the best course of action to take, but Amanda was strongly leaning toward Dr. Michaels's advice.

Even if her tumors had reduced, that still didn't address the reason why she got cancer in the first place (although all of the doctors indicated her early and extensive unprotected sun exposure factored in). She worked tirelessly on coming up with a tailored diet that would specifically address her present needs as well as prevent any more tumors from arising in the future.

Amanda firmly believed that there was an underlying imbalance going on in her body but was hard pressed to find exactly what it was. She did think, however, it was partly to do with her metabolism and immune system, and researched constantly for answers. *Metabolic Typing* was her search tool of that moment, and she did derive a lot of very interesting information from its pages.

In Amanda's Words...

From the point I was healing from back surgeries until the time I was diagnosed with stage-four melanoma cancer, I knew that my body was fighting high toxicity. I believed this was mostly due to the numerous medications I had been prescribed throughout the years following the car accident of 2000. Of course, my health insurance never covered any kind of detoxification therapies. So the toxicity kept building up, I imagine, enough to lower my immune system to the level that it provided cancer with an open door. I am looking into detoxifying my organs through various methods to ease the strain on my immune system so it can fight this.

It has been documented that cancer and other diseases cannot live in an alkalized (oxygenated) environment and that cancer cells commit cell death when pH levels reach 8.0. One of my goals is to bring my pH up to a healthy level. Every time I test myself, I have proven to be extremely acidic, probably, in part, due to the fact that my toxicity level is so high. I have a phone number of a doctor that can do a toxicity test on me, and I think it's important.

Another problem is, although I am eating, I'm basically starving for more food. I seem to be suffering from Cachexia, which is a state of general poor health, malnutrition, weakness, and emaciation. When I eat, I eat a lot, but still often feel hungry afterward. Perhaps it could best be described as a malnourished feeling. This tells me I am depleted in some type of nutrients, minerals, and/or enzymes. But neither the oncologist nor the nutritionist will do tests. I'm not sure who will, but I need to find that type of doctor. I think it's a Naturopath (ND).

Amanda ultimately decided to remain on the Temodar, but she was still searching for a less toxic replacement for the Taxol, with one option being Thalidomide. She made an appointment with a nutritionist/wellness consultant named Trudy who, she learned, performed all the kinds of tests she had been wanting to have done, including food allergy/sensitivity, hair mineral analysis, medical blood work, amino acids/protein deficiencies, DNA/nutritional, hormone imbalance, complete nutritional needs, and metabolism. After these tests were conducted and the results were in, Trudy structured a personal eating plan with an individualized menu for Amanda, which provided her with a lot of hope.

In Amanda's Words...

During my appointment with Trudy, we went over a lot of things, but basically it boils down to this: There are specific tests that I've been wanting to have done to see what "state" my body is in. Upon receiving these findings, we'll gain better insight into exactly how to nourish it with the proper diet and supplements to give me a better chance of recovery. I got a lot of hope from that meeting and look forward to knowing more about the results very soon.

The first test I'm going to get is an Amino Acids Plasma test. It costs a whopping $625— not covered by insurance, of course. It will show what all my levels are of each of the essential amino acids. The second test I need is the Quest Medical Blood Work/CWP Analysis, which might be covered by insurance. I'm just waiting to find out. Otherwise it will be $240.

The third most important test is the Whole Health Food Panel/ALCAT 100. That one is not covered by insurance and is $380. The Organix (Organic Acids) Test is very important but costs $650. However, it will only be accurate after I've been off of chemotherapy for at least a month or two. I am hoping to get it done by December.

After chemo, we went to Wendy, a reflexologist. She began to work on my feet, and I felt instant relief. The worst sore spots on my feet were the same areas that correlate with my lower back, neck, hip, sciatica, where my port is located (probably because it had just been accessed). She definitely freed up some stagnate energy that was in my body. I really felt a major difference. I've had a headache a good majority of today, but that is a common healing reaction when you get bodywork done. In fact, this ties in with a book I'm reading *Hands of Light: Healing Through the Human Energy Field*. I have a real interest in this area and believe it has significant healing potential.

It was getting harder and harder for Amanda to keep up her nutrition. She went through fruit juices like they were going out of style. In fact, she even bought a wheat grass grinder juicer and had a shot of the green stuff every couple of hours. Then came the carrots. Amanda juiced and drank so many that her skin turned orange. I kid you not! While the average person might find humor in that, given the context, it was no laughing matter. If anything, the tremendous extra effort she placed on trying to get well in the face of enormous adversity just demonstrated her extraordinary strength and courage, trying everything possible to reverse this horrible condition.

She was continually on the look out for something…anything that would help her desperate state of affairs. When it became too unbearable for me to watch her vicious struggle, I would just have to go out—anywhere—just out. I didn't want Amanda to see the fear in my eyes. She knew me too well. Even in my despair, my wife put the fight right back in me with a simple wink and a smile. Wow! Can you believe this woman? My God—what *courage!*

Down but Not Out

The tumors were getting more and more painful. The ones on the backs of her legs were starting to press against the skin from underneath, finally ripping it open and breaking through. There were many of these on the backs of her thighs, making it uncomfortable for her to sit. Pillows helped, but then there was the toilet. I managed to get a soft seat for her so the pain would be lessened, and it worked pretty well. Believe me…just the slightest touch on a tumor and bam…pain!

In Amanda's Words…

This past Monday I was scheduled to get chemo, but my white blood cell counts were too low. Dr. Michaels mentioned that he believes the Taxol has basically run its course because I am only stable and not moving forward. For this reason, I filled out paperwork to go on Thalidomide.

I spent tons of time filling out all these questions on this survey for Dr. Gonzalez, and he faxed me back saying he didn't think the vigorous treatment would help me. It's helped other late stage cancer patients, so I don't know how he could think it wouldn't help me, too. I heard he does this with his potential patients first before accepting them to see if they are serious.

My sister, Kristi, and I worked out at her gym Thursday. I got a good sweat going. It felt great. I was able to release some aggression, which also helped some. Then, we went to a vegan deli and had lunch. It was really nice to spend some time with her again, and I'm looking forward to seeing her all this weekend as well.

We had contacted the Cancer Treatment Centers of America, and we were excited that they were going to fly us out to Tulsa, Oklahoma to get treatment. But after checking, Amanda's PPO did not pay enough for them to see her. Considering we paid close to $500 a month for her insurance alone, we were bitterly disappointed by their lack of coverage.

After Dr. Gonzalez denied treating her twice, undoubtedly because he considered Amanda to be too high risk for his trials, she decided to do it on her own with Systemic Enzyme therapy instead of any more chemo. This treatment was said to actually break down the tumors in one's body. The only real danger with it is a strong potential for toxicity. That's why the detoxification part of the regimen and supplementation for the liver and kidneys were so important.

In Amanda's Words…

Well, no luck yet finding a naturopathic doctor or MD with any extensive training in enzyme therapy. Since we would all feel more comfortable, I am searching for a place that will not only administer that type of therapy, but will also monitor my progress so I don't have to "go it alone." I am looking at The International Bio Care in Tijuana, whose protocol includes detoxification, diet, attacking pathogens, hormonal balancing, and rebuilding the immune system.

The 33rd Annual Cancer Convention is being held on September 3rd through 5th in Universal City, California. I really want to go. It's short notice, but I'm going to see if I can work it out. It falls on Saturday, Sunday, and Monday, so Michael will probably have to work. If I'm able to go, I believe it will give me a better idea of where to seek treatment.

The light of hope at the end of the tunnel that I had desperately clung to was rapidly dimming. The next stop was at the office of Dr. Ed McClay of Pacific Oncology & Hematology Associates in Encinitas, California. We were referred to him by our good friends, Bruce and Anat Nilo, the latter of whom was also fighting Stage 4 MM, and drove down as soon as we possibly could. When we finally got there and into an examining room, Amanda looked at me and said, "I love you, Michael Brown… We are together!"

The doctor came in and did a quick examination of Amanda. He asked how she was feeling! "Other than feeling like crap…I'm okay," she said. It made us both chuckle. Amanda loved to hear the way Dr. McClay talked about throwing up as a normal side effect of chemo. He would always refer to it as "yorking." So every time Amanda said she had a bad time and threw up, she would say she "yorked." Then she would laugh at Dr. McClay, and he would laugh right back.

He gave her four options—all completely new to us. Because Amanda was so young, we opted for the newest, most cutting edge treatment called Immunotherapy. But this treatment was truly brutal, and neither Amanda nor I had any idea how tremendously painful it would actually be, despite Dr. McClay's warning. Still, Amanda went through it with consummate strength and dignity. What a woman!

The protocol we decided to pursue required that Amanda have low doses of IL-2 shot directly into all of her sub-q tumors below the skin. The regimen requires an injection in each tumor everyday for two weeks. Combined with Cytoxan, a drug used in the treatment of cancer, the protocol interferes with the multiplication of cancer cells and is supposed to slow or stop their growth and spread in the body.

Dr. McClay claimed to have had an unprecedentedly high success rate with the sub-q's all dying off. He told us that, due to this protocol, he had also seen the body itself learn how to fight the cancer and start attacking other areas below the sub-q level (i.e., in the lungs/brain/liver).

But Amanda needed to stop taking the Temodar a week before initiating this new therapy. She had to stay in San Diego for at least two weeks for daily injections into each of her fourteen sub-q tumors. Although she knew she'd be like a human pincushion, she was willing to try *anything* if there was a possibility it would work. We decided to hold off on any Tijuana clinics until we ran out of other options.

Nearing Baker on the long drive home, Amanda had to relieve herself, so I sped up and pulled into the first fast food place we came to. After assisting her through the front doors, we walked smack into a kid's birthday party. Unfortunately, the bathroom was at the other end of the dining room, and as I held her arm so she could walk the distance, I heard the "ews" and "yuks" emitting from the children's table as they stared and pointed at the ugly, black sores that marred her delicate beauty. On our way out, one little girl screeched, "Mommy...what's *that* on her face?"

I didn't say a word, but after I'd closed both of our car doors, I helplessly turned to my wife. She simply shrugged and said, "Kids will be kids." Then she smiled weakly, and I drove on, thinking, *Dear Lord, I am so blessed.* There was just no one else who could possibly compare.

In Amanda's Words...

We spent some quality time with good friends yesterday and took a dip in their pool in Vegas. After making our plane and hotel reservations and arranging Michael's schedule for my two-week-long stay in San Diego, we were informed that my insurance would only pay half the cost for this treatment since Dr. McClay was considered out of my network. We're going through with it anyway, as we both believe it's the best thing to do.

In addition to the Immunotherapy, I have added two other things to my protocol, personalizing it to give my body the best chance it can have to overcome this condition. As soon as they arrive, I will be adding cesium/potassium to raise my pH and three to five cups per day of tea made from common birch tree (Betula alba) to my other daily supplements. Research indicates that the Betulinic acid in the powder on the bark dissolves multiple melanoma cell lines and also keeps the cancer from returning. These three treatments have given me high hopes.

Michael gave me a full-body check yesterday and found about fifteen more sub-q (just under the skin) tumors, which brings them up to about thirty now. This morning before my appointment, he'll mark each of them with a pen.

Dr. McClay injected about half the tumors, only the ones that were big enough to receive an injection, and said we should just watch the smaller ones for now.

The injections on the top of my head hurt the most. He explained that there were more nerves up there and, boy, did I feel every single one of them! About an hour after these injections, I got a huge hot flash, and my breathing quickened. All of a sudden, I started to feel as if I was going to blackout and got real sweaty.

I was picking up some medication for Amanda when I got her call. She was mumbling, "Help...help!" in a barely audible voice. I rushed back to the hotel and, when I arrived, found her shaking uncontrollably with extreme chills. When that subsided, she was still extremely cold, so I got her straight into the bath. Although that helped to warm her up, her temperature was still low at 97.3 degrees.

During the course of the evening, her temperature continued to rise until it reached 100.3. Although Dr. McClay had warned us this was an inevitable side effect of the treatment, he also told Amanda that she shouldn't take the extra strength Tylenol he had prescribed until her temperature reached 102 degrees. However, because we didn't have a thermometer handy and, hence, didn't know her actual temperature, she took it too soon. As such, it had little effect. She just instinctively reached for relief when the horrible feelings first came on.

In Amanda's Words...

The results of the scans that I had done on Friday came back, and we reviewed them with Dr. McClay. My brain MRI seemed encouraging, as it picked up only three tumors. Previously, they had radiated six with the Gamma Knife, so it appears there is a reduction in the other three. However, the scanner skips .2 mm after every .5 mm of scan, so I'm thinking very small ones could have been missed.

Although the lesion in the right temporal lobe shows ring-like enhancement, the doctor said we don't have to treat it immediately because it is so small. We are hoping that these injections into the sub-q tumors will trigger my immune system to attack the tumors in my brain and throughout the rest of my body.

Dr. McClay asked me to stop taking the birch tea for now to see if the therapy works on its own. He wants to make sure that it doesn't cancel out the immunotherapy, as is sometimes the case, but he said it was fine for me to continue the cesium/potassium.

Please send up prayers to heaven that this new immunotherapy treatment will rid my body of melanoma once and for all.

Photographs

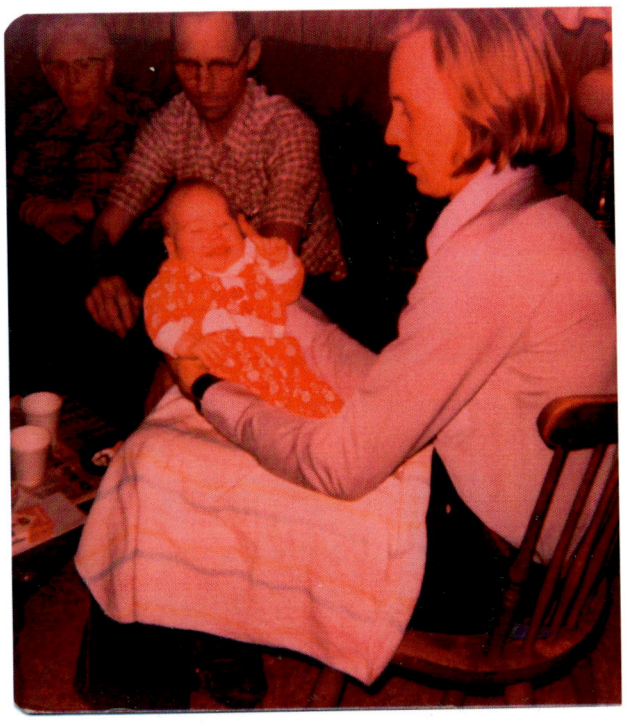

Amanda being held by father, Dwight,
Grandpa Welton in the back ground

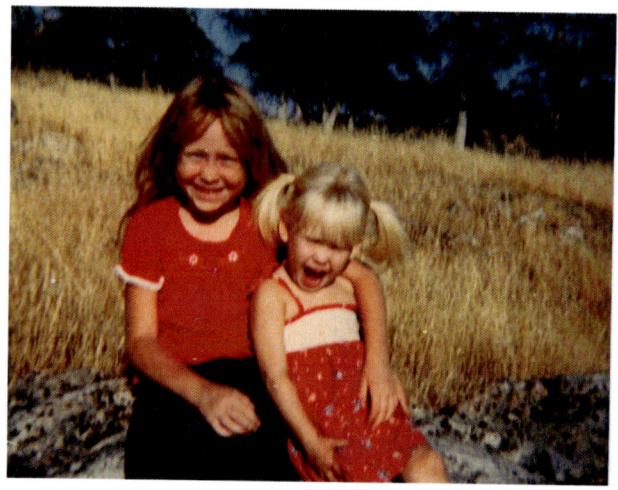

Amanda and Kristi playing outside their home

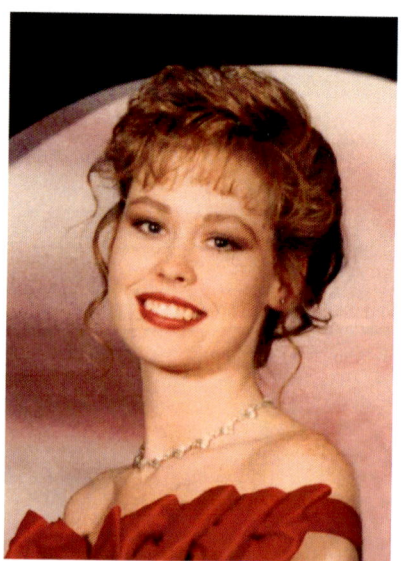

Prom

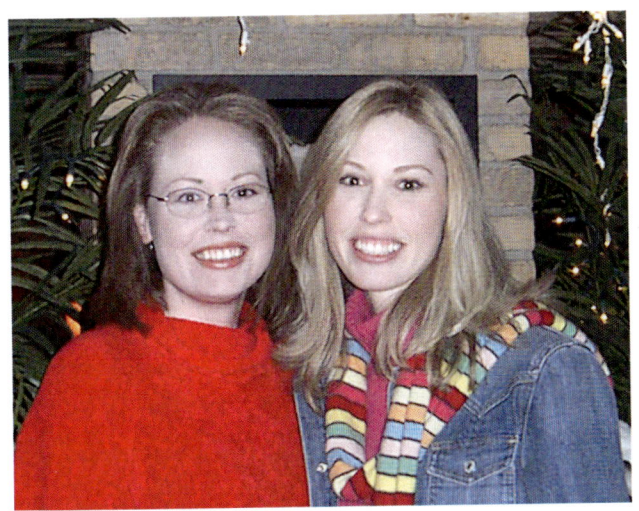

Amanda and Kristi

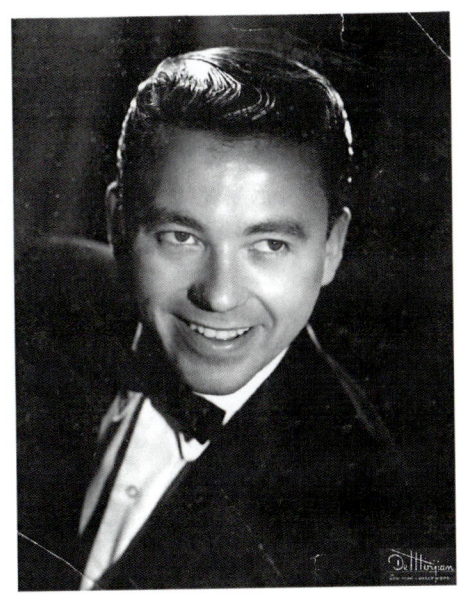

My Father, Ronnie Brown

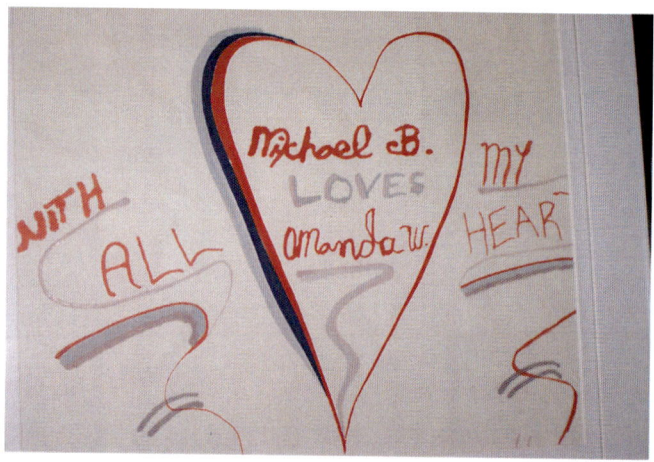

Picture I painted for Amanda. July 4th, Lake Tahoe

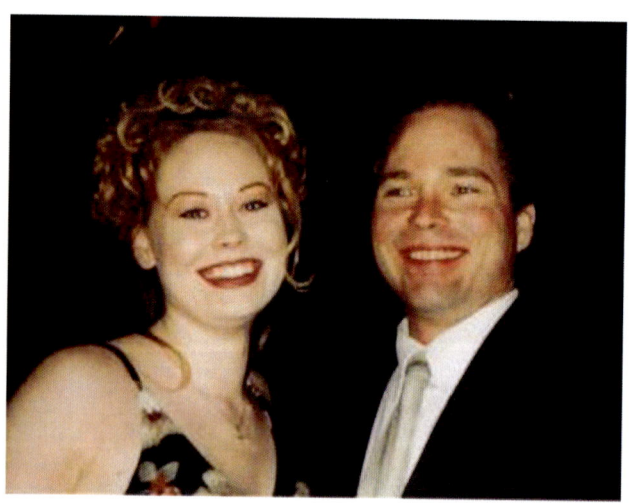

Taken right after I asked Amanda to marry me

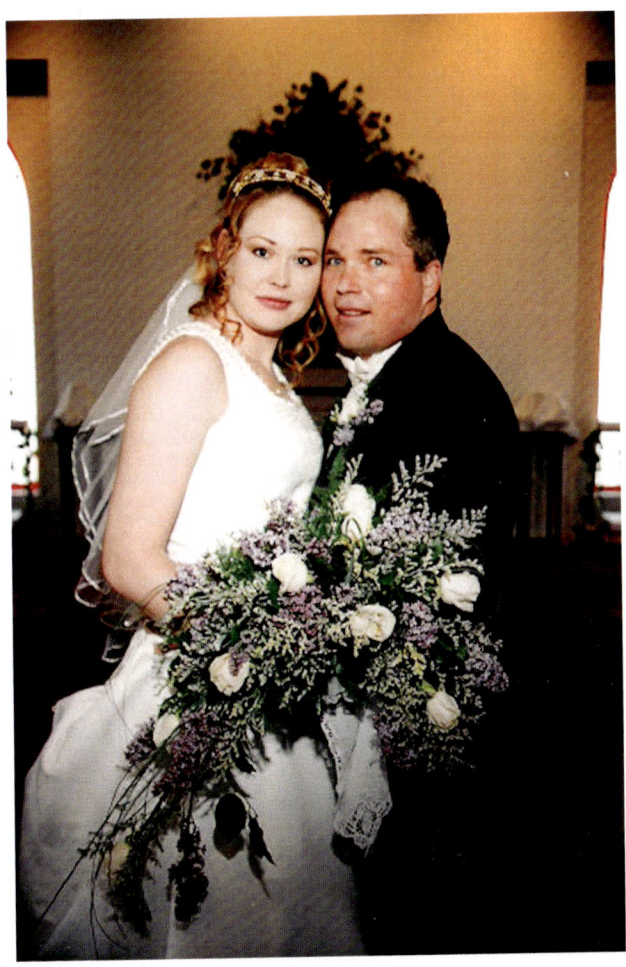

Our wedding

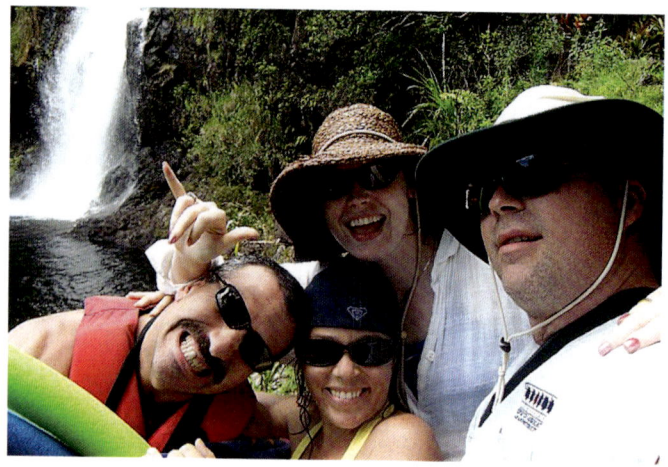

Scott, Shari, Amanda, and myself at our waterfall

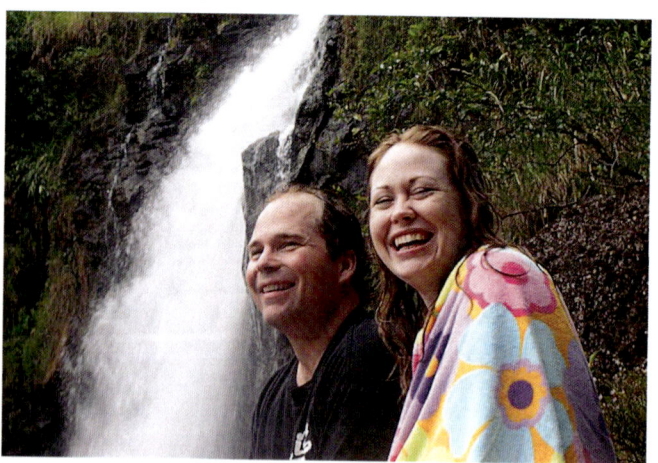

Enjoying our view high up the cliff from our waterfall

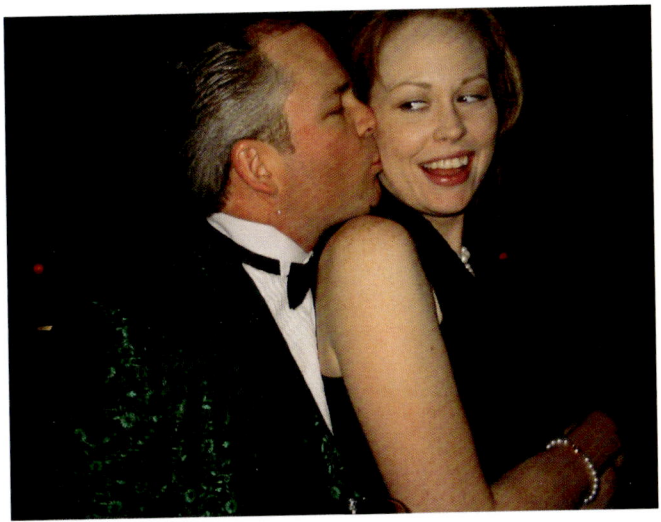

Giving my beautiful wife a kiss

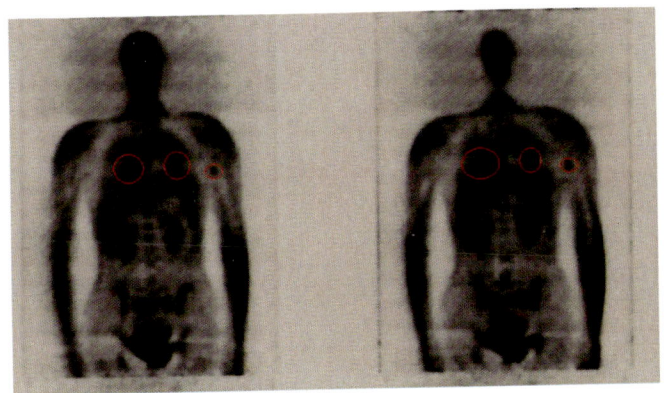

CAT scan of Amanda's lungs

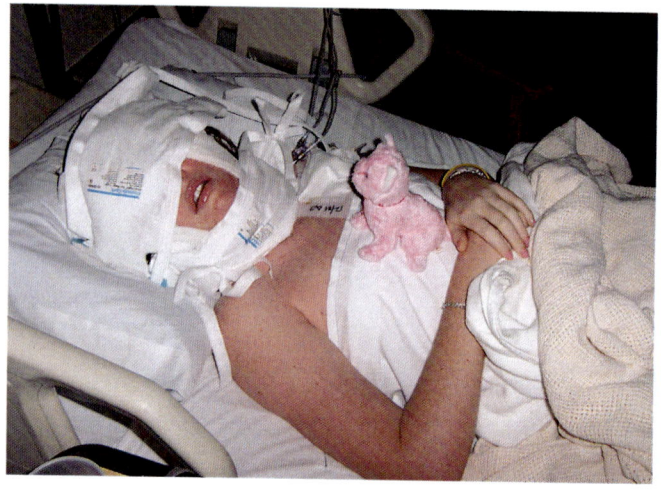

Moments after Amanda's biochemo treatment

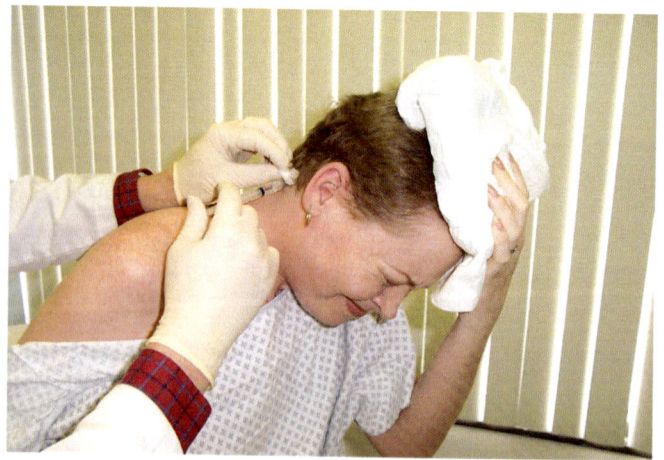

Immunotherapy treatment

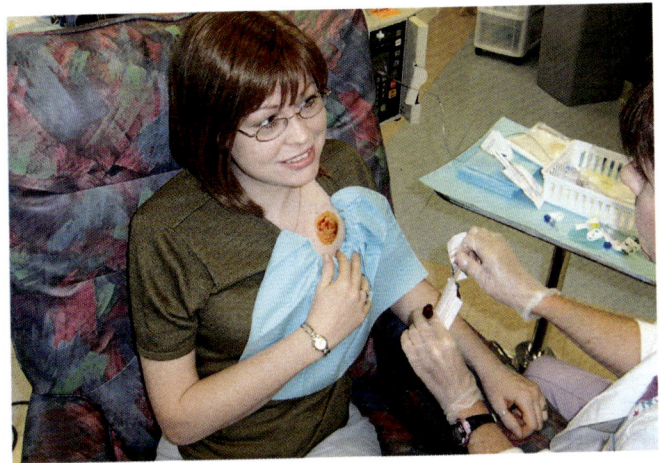

Taxol infusion

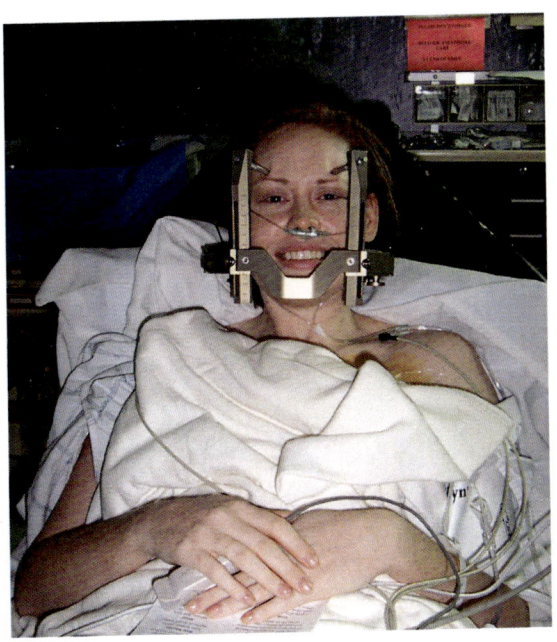

Smiling through it all

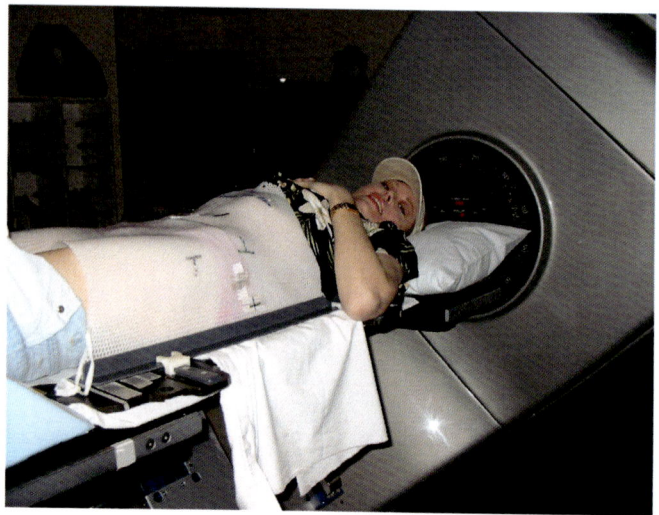

Body radiation

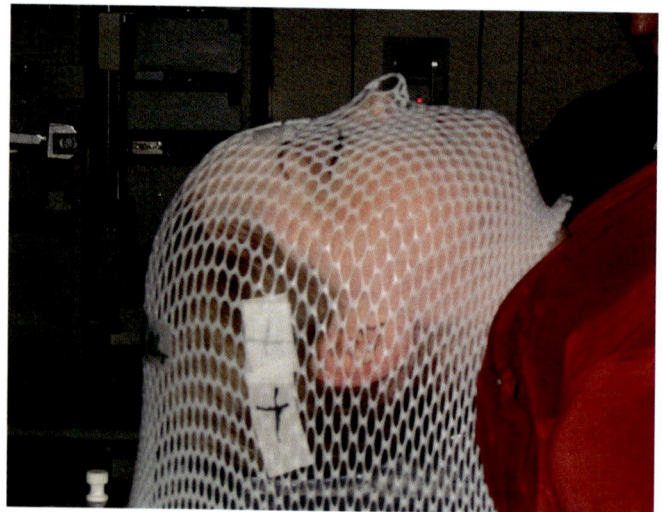

Brain radiation

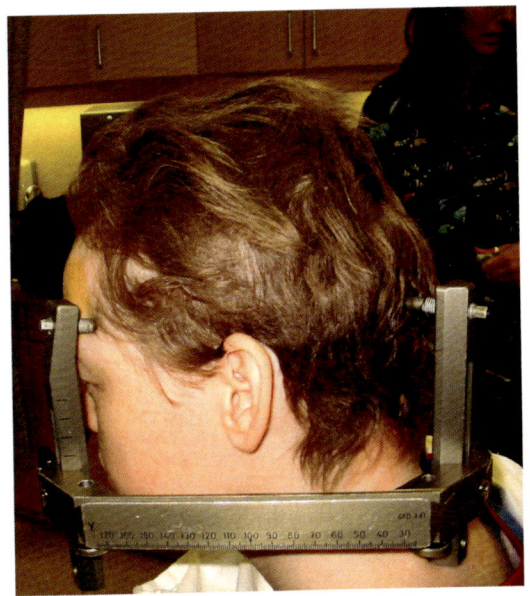

Gamma knife treatment

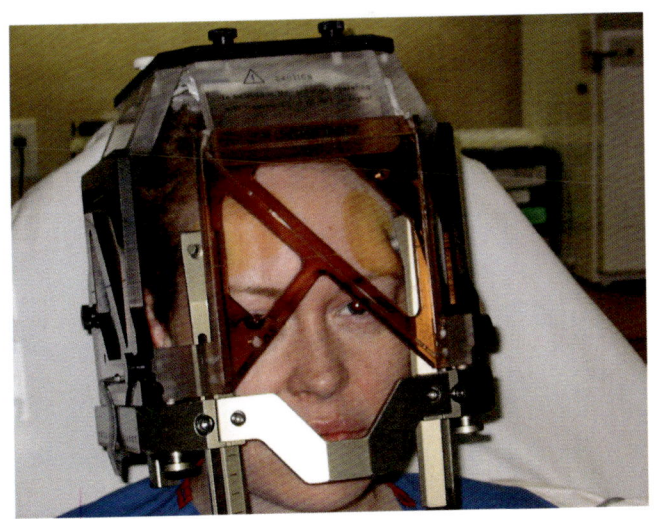

Gamma knife treatment

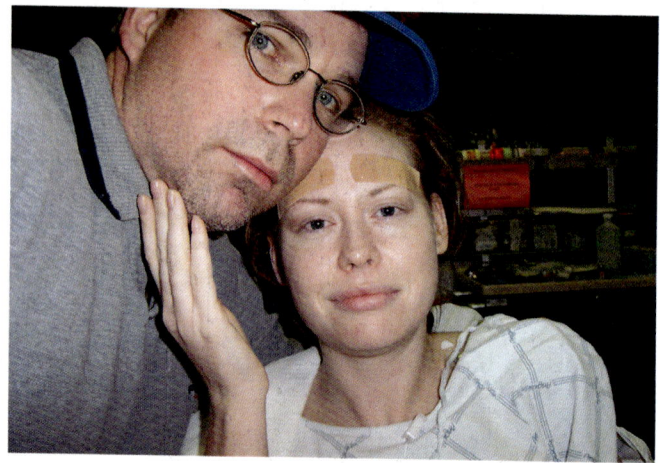

Taken after gamma knife treatment

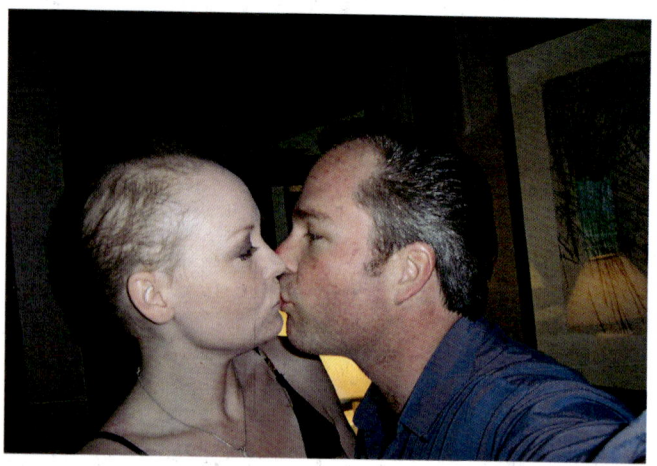

Loving my beautiful wife

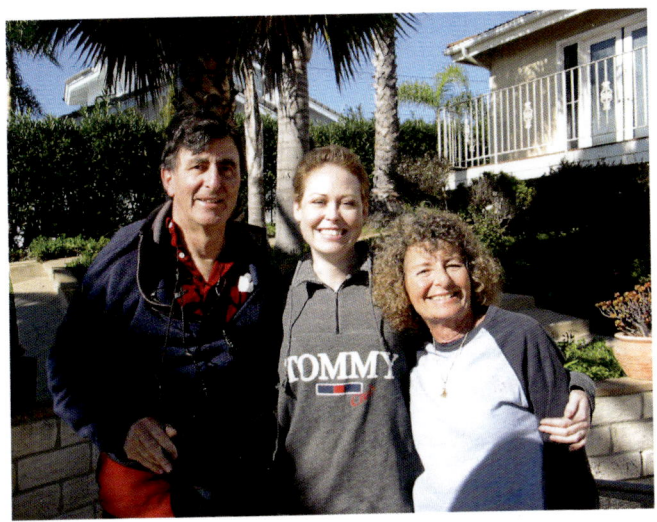

Our dear friends, Paul and Roberta Kaplan

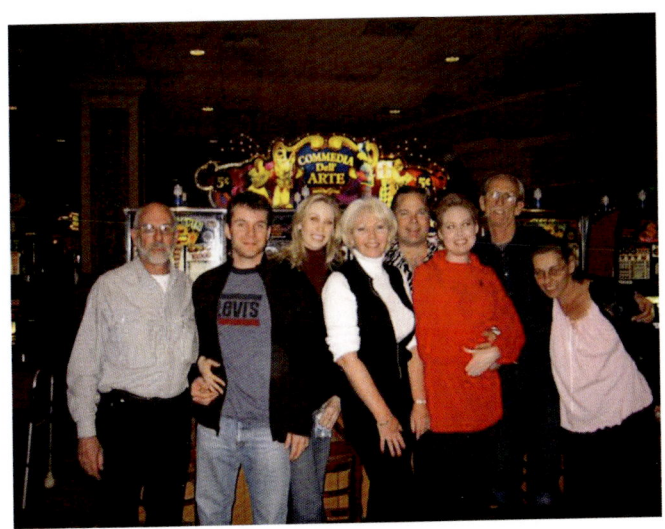

The family

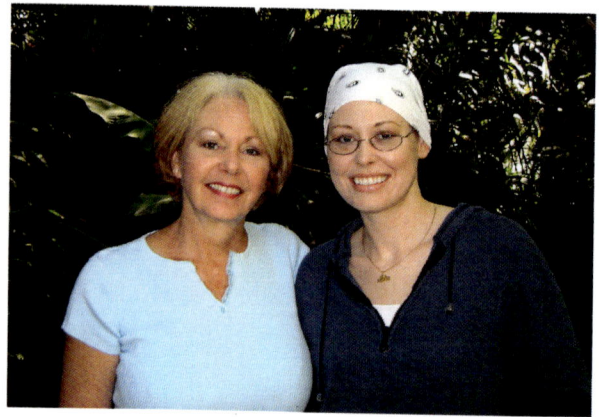

Amanda and her mother, Connie

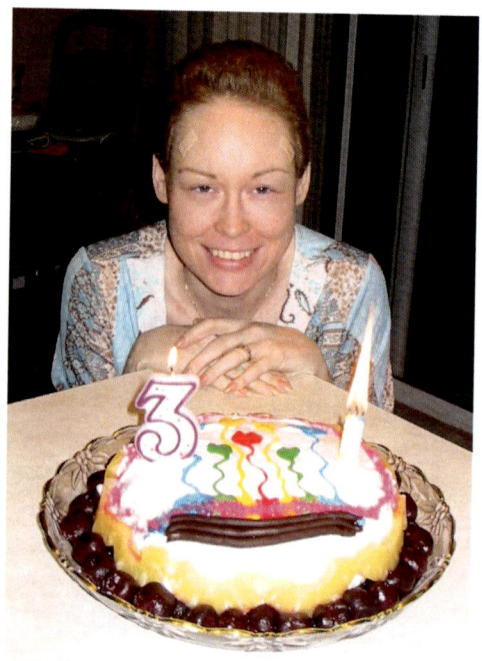

Amanda's 31st birthday cake I made her

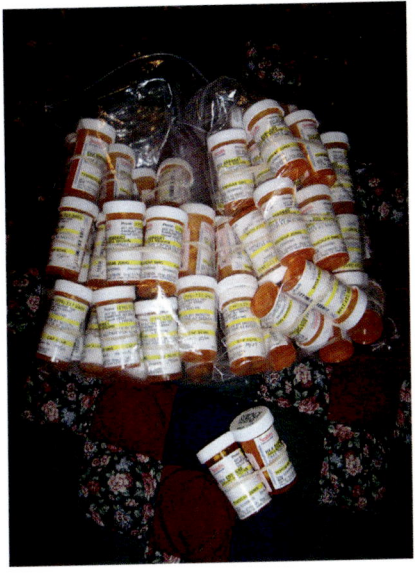

This is just one prescription pick up from the pharmacy

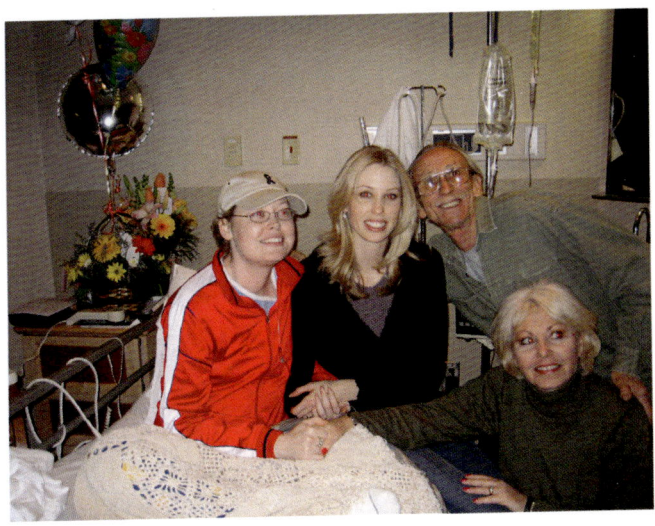

Amanda's family surrounding her bedside before brain surgery

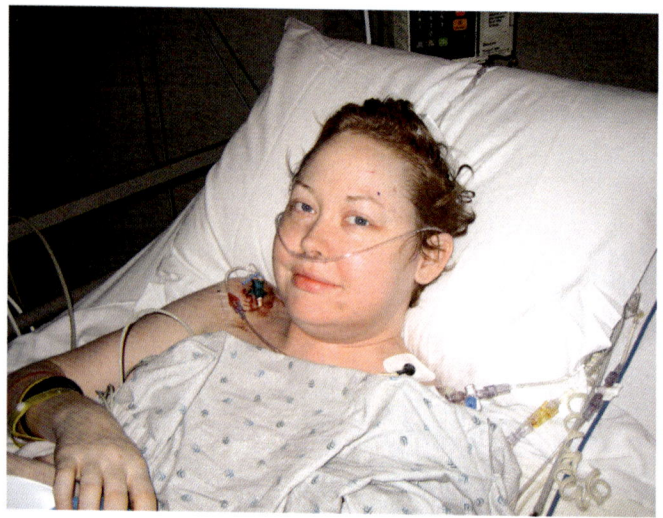

Waiting for brain surgery

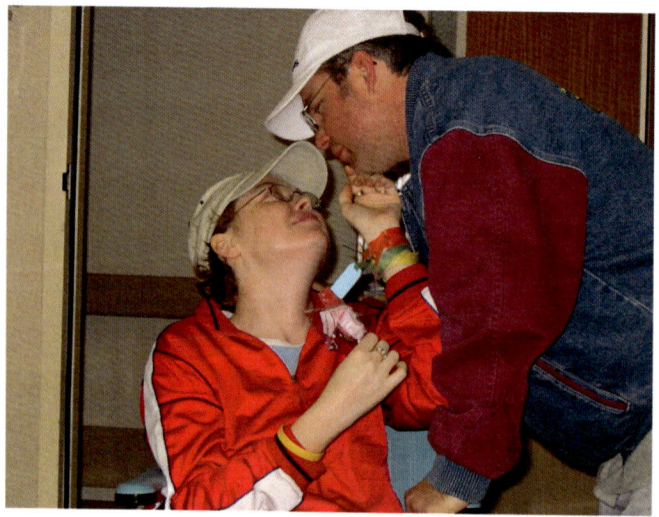

Ready to take my wife home after her brain operation

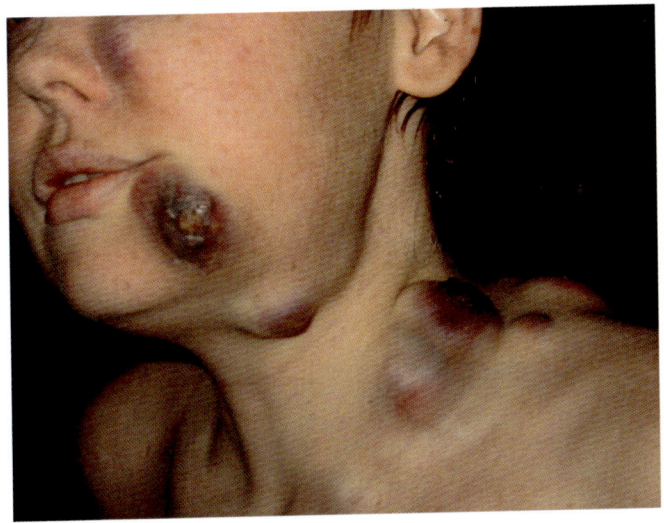

Melanomas devastating effects

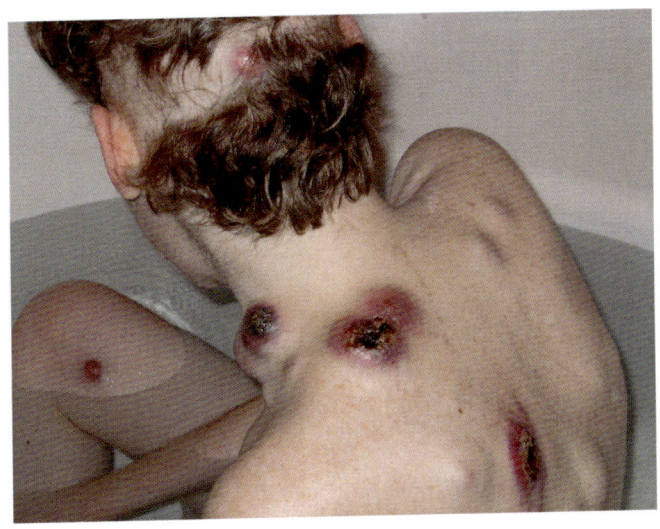

Amanda doing her best to live a normal life

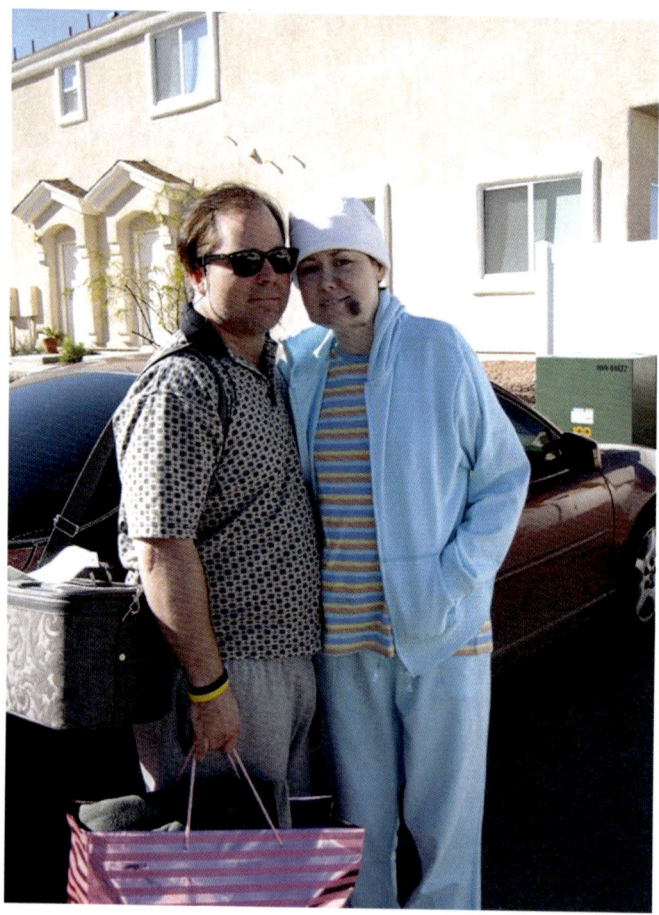

Our last trip down to Orange County to try a new treatment

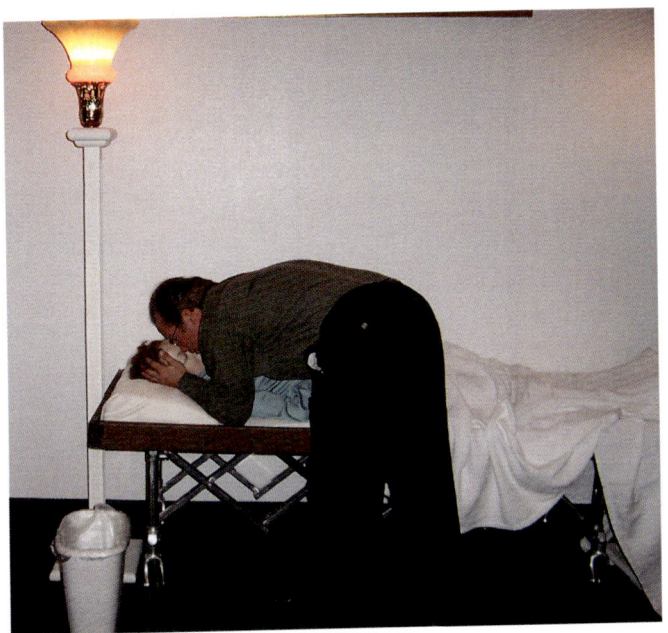

My last kiss

First Response

At Amanda's next appointment with Dr. McClay, he told her that she was a "quick responder" and was very pleased at her body's reaction to the IL-2 treatment. And although she'd felt like she'd been walking in the dark with death on her doorstep for the past year, she was finally starting to see a light at the end of the tunnel. In fact, Dr. McClay was very optimistic that she could achieve complete remission, or NED (no evidence of disease), soon after this series of treatment ended.

While we were naturally overjoyed at the news, it did seem almost too good to be true. However, the doctor explained that even though he had been injecting sub-q melanoma tumors for twenty years to date, he had only been doing so in patients who had sub-q, and not deeper tissue tumors. But the strategy he was using on Amanda was to inject the sub-q tumors directly with IL-2, which is naturally manufactured by the body to attack a virus/invader. Sadly, because melanoma has a way of cloaking itself from this normal defense mechanism, it is not recognized as "bad," and the body doesn't try to defend itself from it. Therefore, IL-2 is not usually manufactured in response to a melanoma invasion. Dr. McClay's new method of treatment was to inject the reachable tumors directly with IL-2, which would then go to work fighting the invader. As a result, it was hoped that the body would subsequently learn that melanoma is, in fact, an enemy that needs to be destroyed.

Doctor McClay told us about his first success with this treatment. Like Amanda, his patient had sub-q *and* deep metastatic tumors. Due to their depth and location, he was unable to inject them with IL-2 and only injected her sub-q tumors. After nine days of injections, her body had time to recognize melanoma as an enemy and manufacture its own IL-2 as a normal defense response. All—I repeat—*all* of her tumors vanished. Her body came to understand that melanoma was a formidable foe, which needed to be aggressively battled.

She was soon declared NED—melanoma free! Three years later she developed a single reoccurrence and immediately returned to Dr. McClay. He administered the same treatment, but that round only required three days of injections before her system once again responded and fought back. That was two years earlier, and she remained NED.

Amanda was only the second person to be so treated, and Dr. McClay chose fifteen of her sub-qs, which were close to the surface, as the "training tumors." He injected them with IL-2 and believed her body would also learn that there was a "hiding invader" and begin manufacturing its own IL-2 to continue the combat.

Within the first few days of treatment, she had a great deal of pain in the injected and non-injected tumors (in her lungs and other areas). But by day four, Dr. McClay decided not to reinject several of her sub-qs because they had become too small. You can just imagine our delight! The tumors began to flatten out and appeared red and angry—kind of like an infected cut would look. Amanda also believed her deeper tumors were also beginning to be attacked.

Over the previous several months, she had been told by various doctors that she'd have to be on chemo for the rest of her life. Several of them even gave her actual timeframes as to how long (not very) she might survive. And now, Dr. McClay was assuring her that her body could fight this killer disease. It only needed to be trained to detect the enemy. We were honestly afraid to believe it might be true.

Now bear in mind, as previously stated, these treatments were no walk in the park. They caused severe chills, which lasted about an hour, and then her fever would continue to climb, often exceeding 104 degrees. It was constant rounds of hot baths for the chills followed by ice packs for the fevers. She was also, very unfortunately, in the 20 to 30 percent of patients who developed a histamine rash all over her body, which *really* itched. Dr. McClay prescribed Benedryl and Atarax to control these symptoms. In spite of it all, Amanda was excited with her progress but was continually exhausted from the raging war going on inside her.

In Amanda's Words...

A lot has changed since my last post. I lost a very dear friend of mine, Anat, on the 25th to melanoma. We met her at the John Wayne Cancer Institute and clicked immediately. Over the course of the last year, since our mutual diagnosis, we had been fighting side by side. She had a heart of gold and will be sorely missed by many people.

I have an itchy feeling in various places all over, mostly at previous injection sites like my scalp. This tells me that there is still IL-2 in my body. Since I haven't had an injection in a while, I must be manufacturing my own. I pray that my body has learned to recognize melanoma as the enemy and will continue its attack on these tumor cells. One spot on my right hip, which received an injection, is healing nicely and is actually pushing the small tumor through my skin to the surface. It's wonderful to see one of these bastards come out of my body and die. Although only time will tell, we are hopeful that I am on the right track for a full recovery.

Another bit of satisfying news: The Nevada Equal Rights Commission found in our favor and ruled that my employer did, in fact, discriminate against me. They did not accommodate my disability as required by law.

A short time later, I performed a full body check on Amanda, noting where all of her tumors were. It was terrifying because there were so many new ones, and I called Dr. McClay out of concern for their sheer *numbers*. These new ones actually hurt her too, unlike the ones previously treated. He said that if they hurt, it was a good sign, as it indicated there was an immune response taking place. Otherwise, they would not be hurting. All the tumors that he had injected over the past weeks were now rock-hard, like actual pebbles under her skin. However, he assured us that this was also a good sign, because the tumors were becoming fibrous and would eventually disappear.

In Amanda's Words...

I'm worried and think it's time for some more "nontraditional" treatment. As soon as we have radiated the tumor in my spinal canal and it goes away, I plan to get another round of Immunotherapy. The last treatment caused it to swell so much that I had an unbearable amount of pain down my entire right leg, and I cannot go through that again. I handle pain better than most, I believe, but that was too much. Still, I'll continue to do anything possible to help my body fight this damn disease!

I have decided to write a book about all my life experiences, including my back injury/surgeries and the cancer saga in particular. I had been thinking about this for many months, but just the other day I mentioned it to Michael for the first time. Saying it out loud (especially since it was to my husband) somehow made it real. Immediately, I got the feeling that it is the Lord's will for me to do so. Also, I desperately need life goals other than just beating this unspeakably cruel disease. People keep telling me how inspirational I am. If I put it all in a book, I might be able to inspire even more people that really need it. I think I have quite a story to share and hope that other people, especially other cancer patients, can benefit from my experiences. So, with that in mind, I will work on the book at least a little bit every day until it is finished. The idea of becoming a published author is quite intriguing to both Michael and me. It gives me one more thing to look forward to.

Emergency Intervention

In mid-November of 2005, Amanda started treatment with Dr. Royal at New Hope Medical in Las Vegas. He and his partner, Dr. Friesen, were working on a regimen of therapies to help get her immune system up and running again. He looked shocked when he examined her because of the extensiveness of the disease and, frankly, by the fact she was still alive. When she asked him if he had had any previous patients with her degree of cancer, he replied "No, because they never make it this long." Of course, he hurriedly added that she was an encouraging exception to the rule.

The doctor told my wife, in a nutshell, that her immune system and organs (in particular her adrenal glands, liver, and kidneys) were on the verge of breaking down, and she needed emergency immunology interventional treatment. He immediately prescribed a daily infusion of amino acids, minerals, and estrogen, which she started right away.

In addition, she began a regimen of oral supplements, including Poly-MVA (a combination of minerals, vitamins and amino acids), Maitake D Fraction (maitake mushroom extract to support the immune system), acid/alkalines, ImmPower (which maintains peak natural killer cell function), Pregnenolone, and DHEA.

Unfortunately, New Hope Medical treatments were not covered by medical insurance (with the exception of normal blood-work-type tests), and payment was due at time of service. That day's bill alone was a whopping $942.98. This included the initial consult with Dr. Royal, a sixty-day supply of supplements, and an infusion, with the former averaging $135 each, which she needed every day for at least a month.

By this time, my usual morning routine went something like this: I'd wake up, go find Amanda, wrap her arms around me and receive my soothing rush of love. This morning I found her in the kitchen, wearing my blue robe. She opened the robe and wrapped it around the two of us. I held her close, and we danced for a minute on the tile floor.

Less than an hour later while writing in her notebook, Amanda suddenly looked up at me with pure terror in her eyes and said. "I don't feel well, and I can't write... it's going down. I can't comprehend the words and how they're spelled." Panic stricken, I helped her into the bedroom, but she was feeling so woozy and nauseated, we went to the bathroom where I sat her down on the toilet with me next to her on the side of the tub.

She put her hands on her face and started crying, "Something's wrong...something's wrong!" I turned my head to get a towel to wipe her tears and heard what sounded like a snort...and then another back-to-back. When I turned around to face her, Amanda's body was in a full convulsion. Her head started to rise up and then turned to her right side. I screamed, "Amanda!" and grabbed her.

Although I tried to get her to the bed, her legs were dragging behind me like dead weight. I therefore laid her down on the bedroom floor where she began to gasp for air and foam at the mouth. I immediately searched for something to prevent her from biting her tongue but was too late. A mixture of blood and foam spewed from her mouth like a fountain. Although frozen with fear, I managed to turn her on her side so she wouldn't choke on the fluids. A few minutes later (which seemed like an eternity), the seizure was starting to subside, but her eyes were completely dark—no color at all. She was dazed; however, I was able to get her up and onto the bed. She said, "What's happening?"

I said, "Just lay down...don't move, honey!"

I ran to the phone and called 911. Thankfully, they responded very quickly. After meeting them at the door, I led them in the direction of the bedroom where we discovered Amanda coming down the hallway. I grabbed her and put her down on the couch. Her head turned to the right, and she couldn't feel anything.

I cried out to her, "Amanda.... Amanda...can you hear me? Amanda!"

She turned her head toward me every time I said her name. But then her head would slowly turn down to her right side again. The paramedic told me she was still having seizures. Her head turned so very far to the right it would have had to hurt her neck if, in fact, she could feel anything. Just then, another seizure began. All I could do was stand there with my mouth open. The paramedics said there was nothing to be done until it stopped. While we were waiting it out, I called Amanda's mother to tell her what was happening. I'm sure I wasn't speaking too clearly, and there was a lot of static on my cell phone, so all my poor mother-in-law could understand was that there was something wrong with her daughter. I can't imagine how frightened she must have been.

Amanda's father happened to be driving by and saw the ambulance at our house. When he came through the door, he was absolutely horrified to see what was going on. After we got her into the ambulance, she started to convulse once more so violently that the paramedics couldn't even hold her down. She started crying and screaming at the same time, and although it sounded like she was trying to say something, the words were just gibberish.

I could barely speak myself but managed to whisper, "It's okay, Amanda. I'm right here. I'm right here, honey!" She calmed down for just a moment, so I kept talking to her.

As the ambulance pulled away, I got into my car and, as a former amateur race car driver, employed the full benefit of my experience, passing every other vehicle on the road, to get to the hospital in Las Vegas by the time she arrived. When I got there, the ambulance driver told me they had given her some medication and she had finally calmed down. "I'm so very sorry, Mr. Brown," he said with great feeling in his voice. I was touched by this one of many everyday heroes we encountered along our desperate journey.

Bread and Butter

Whenever Amanda and I would walk together, we always held hands. If something got between us and we had to temporarily break our connection, Amanda would call out two words that went together, like, "peanut butter and jelly," "pork chops and apple sauce," or, most frequently, "bread and butter." I would make fun by saying two words that didn't go together, like "sardines and chocolate milk." She would lovingly squeeze my arm, and I couldn't have adored it more.

As the days went by, Amanda continued to fail. By late November, she could hardly stand and had no feeling in the major part of the lower half of her body. Due to the tumors, she could only lie on her left side. They were so painful, she cried out in the middle of her sleep. And yet, she kept right on fighting with all of her might each and every moment. We tried to remain strong, but overwhelming fear was our constant companion.

However, a short time later, a bright star shot through the darkness of our never-ending night when, after my performance at the Forty Deuce, I was summoned to the VIP booth at the request of singer Josh Groban. He wanted to tell me how much he enjoyed the show and bought me a rum and coke. I don't remember how the conversation got started, but I began to tell him about Amanda. After we finished our drink, he hugged me and asked for my cell number. I walked away, thinking to myself, *Josh Groban is one of the nicest, kindest celebs I have ever met.*

A couple of days later, while playing a private party at Sam's Town Casino, my cell phone rang backstage. Picking up, I was greeted with the words, "Hello, Michael? This Josh Groban." I was speechless. He proceeded to ask me for my home number so he could speak with Amanda. Shakily, I relayed it to him and thanked him from the bottom of my heart. As I hung up, I immediately called home to tell Amanda that Josh Groban was going to call her, and she excitedly replied, "Yeah...I know. He's on the other line!" I quickly laughed and hung up the phone so she could continue her conversation with Josh. A most touching gesture from a truly wonderful man.

In Amanda's Words...

Recently, I've realized a few things; primarily that, more and more, I try not to express the extraordinary terror I have in facing this challenge. For instance, one minute I am crying my eyes out to my husband. The next minute, I am on the phone speaking with someone I care about, and I instantly sound happy, like I don't have a care in the world.

I probably do this to spare other people's feelings. I think I now believe there is enough tragedy in life that surely others don't have to continually share in mine.

I did the same thing when I went through my back surgeries. I think that's why a lot of people thought I was feigning pain; though, of course, it was always damn near unbearable.

I suppose I could be one of the best actresses in Hollywood, smiling merrily through all of the devastation. I paint everything in brilliant happy colors, while inside I am totally broken, my soul curled up in the fetal position, begging for relief.

I cannot and will not allow many people to see this side of me, even though it is there. God gives me a huge amount of strength and comfort, as does my husband. But even with that, I still desperately need to vent at times.

I've been feeling very frustrated for a while now. When I feel like this, crying and voicing my concerns makes me feel better about things. I am grateful that I am alive, and this experience has taught me to value every single moment. You never know when a day may be your last...none of us do, whether or not we have been diagnosed with a terminal disease.

I have several recent concerns. For one thing, I am unsure about how my condition is progressing. I need to talk again with Dr. McClay. I am worried because there are so many new tumors popping up. The ones that were injected are all rock hard but don't seem to be dissipating fast enough.

I need to get scans done again before I can undergo any more injections because I am afraid they will bring on more tumors, in addition to being extremely painful. The fact is, each time I have gotten injections, I have had more tumors surface almost immediately afterward. My body is feeling like it's at maximum capacity for fighting my tumor load already. I simply don't want to provoke any more disease to surface until my body has had time to get rid of what has already been treated.

Lately, I think that one of two things is happening: either my body is starting to fight off these tumors, or the cancer is taking over. It is hard to tell which, but I pray I am starting to get better. I'm not certain, however, which of these hypotheses is true. That's why I need more scans.

My other concern is that my doctors, whose opinions I truly value, simply disagree on administering Estron to me. Dr. Royal believes that it will help stop the growth of melanoma, but Dr. McClay is skeptical and asked to see some of his studies indicating that pure Estron could demonstrate some efficacy in battling the cancer. He thinks both think Dr. Royal is basing his opinion on synthetic Estrogen and/or In vitro results instead of In vivo.

At this point, not being a trained medical researcher, I don't know what to believe or how to make a reasonable decision if I have to.

Actually, I just want to get better, and when my doctors don't agree, it just compounds the problem. They never said that combining conventional and homeopathic medicine would be easy!

Tonight I broke down in tears to Michael. This was far from the first time I had done this, and I'm sure far from the last. I am strong most of the time but, as my Mom pointed out, "only human." For me, crying is a major stress reliever. It helped me through my back surgeries as well as the long healing time that followed. And it has helped me through the first year of fighting with this horrendous disease.

I know my pain and crying hurts Michael and raises his blood pressure. After all, the most he can really do during my worst moments is hold me and pray. Clearly, all this drama affects his health, so I try my best to keep it from him and cry in private when I have to. Sometimes, though, this is not an option for me, and I have to reach out to him. It's a catch-22, because we are both under an enormous amount of stress.

It's unbelievable what he goes through as my sole provider and full time caretaker. My poor husband sleeps in shifts, if he's lucky and the phone doesn't ring. Right now, he's suffering from moderate hypertension and recently had to go on a new blood pressure medication to control it.

We could not afford to add him to my Cobra policy, and he currently has no insurance. He is waiting on a contract renewal at work and then, hopefully, insurance will be provided, but that could take some time. Yes, his health is worrisome to me. He just checked into getting more life insurance for himself "just in case."

This disease has not only affected me in every way, but Michael's health is being sacrificed as well. He witnesses first-hand all the frustration, anger, pain, and increasingly frequent breakdowns that I experience.

I am able to hide my suffering fairly well in front of most people, but it's real difficult to hide my feelings from my husband. He knows me too well.

Personally, I am such an empathetic person that I can sense someone's worry just by hearing their tone of voice. If I know I am the direct cause of that worry, it hurts me, especially in the case of that person being the one I love more than anything in this world. I don't want to be a burden to any of my loved ones.

A few months back I even started a separate page in the website just to note my pain, so it wasn't part of the latest update anymore. I thought this could be a way for me to vent, which, as I have indicated before, seems to make me feel a bit better. With this "pain page," I can do so without parading my suffering in front of my husband or family. Besides, most people who check out my website usually just read the latest update. Hiding my pain to spare everyone's feelings takes a lot of energy—unfortunately, more than I have right now.

Dealing with the world with regard to my suffering is a fine line I've been walking for quite some time. I have come to the conclusion, though, that, as difficult as it is to see, hear about, or read, this is my truth! It's my reality.

I am not ashamed of my scars or what I am going through. I feel it is my duty to expose the raw truth of this journey and share my experiences with other cancer patients and caregivers around the world.

Another Round

The day after she made the above entry, Amanda suffered two more seizures. As it was during the afternoon, I was right there when it happened, and after calling 911, all I could do was hold her in my arms while we waited for the ambulance to arrive. She was taken to Southern Hills Hospital and had a CAT scan later that night. It turned out she had a brain hemorrhage, possibly from last month's gamma knife procedure. The doctors said it was critical and that they needed to get her to Sunrise Hospital in Vegas where they could perform surgery if needed.

After her first Gamma Knife treatment, Amanda had another dream. This time she loved it.

It was early in the morning around 5am. She awoke with a huge smile on her face. She nudged me to get up and she began to tell me what she had just dreamt.

She was walking in a stream that was literally crystal clear. She was holding Jesus' hand. He was in pure white. She noticed his feet were not getting wet as he was walking on top of the water. She couldn't explain to me the amount of joy and happiness she felt. She said there was a lake that was the most beautiful lake she'd ever seen; she was able to see everything on the bottom of the lake as well as on the top, pure as can be. She said she saw me in this lake as if I was waiting for her to come over.

When she told me her dream, she did it quickly. Then she said she was trying to go back to sleep quickly so she could try and get back to that same dream.

In Amanda's Words...

Well, we received some news about what treatment I will pursue next. We're a bit disappointed that my immune system doesn't seem to be strong enough right now to withstand more IL-2 Immunotherapy injections. Still, I am relieved because they are so excruciatingly painful each time. After all I just went through with the brain seizures and hemorrhages, my body is in strong need of rest and recuperation.

Dr. McClay wants to wean me off of the steroids I was given to combat the swelling in my brain before he attempts another round of IL-2 injections. He says the steroids could pull the immune system down to nothing if I stay on them. Obviously, we need it to be in tip-top shape. The hope is that my body will retain a memory of how to get rid of these tumors through immunotherapy treatments.

While I am weaning myself off of these steroids over the next six weeks, we've decided to go back on Chemo just long enough for my immune system to get back to speed. In this manner, I will still be fighting the cancer in some way.

We'll drive back to Vegas/Pahrump on Wednesday where we will start on the Triple T Treatment: Temodar, Thalidomide, and Taxotere. Temodar and Thalidomide are pills, and the Taxotere is a once-a-week infusion. Dr. McClay was very insistent that I remain on the immune-system-building regimen with Dr. Royal in Vegas. Basically, Dr. McClay stressed that the immune system needs to be fully empowered in order for the immunotherapy to be effective. So, we are in a race to boost mine.

I had a PET scan this afternoon. We're going to get the results tomorrow morning when we go back to Dr. McClay's. We hope and pray that the lung tumors have shrunk. Also, we dropped off my recent MRI scans with the brain hemorrhages to the Gamma Knife doctor at Scripts Hospital in San Diego. He'll call us on our drive tomorrow and let us know if they were due to the radiated tumor or a new tumor, which bled and has not yet been treated. The physicians at Sunrise Hospital in Vegas thought it was from my last two Gamma Knife procedures. My October MRI scans only showed one tumor, not two.

Happily, we're planning to meet with some dear friends, Paul and Roberta, for breakfast tomorrow. They are from Carlsbad and are in the fight against cancer as well. They are such a fantastically lovely couple, so goodhearted and caring. They give me hope and encouragement through their own victories. I need that strength to keep up this supreme struggle. We've been very blessed to meet them both.

After we visit with our wonderful friends, Michael is going to take me to Sea World for a little fun and a break from our daily grind. We both enjoy sea animals, so I'm sure it will be a fun and relaxing time for both of us. It will be during the week, too, so it shouldn't be very busy, which will be nice. Of course, we'll take pictures to capture our experiences!

If there's one major thing this is teaching me, it's to live your life to the fullest and cherish every moment you are blessed with. Life is so very, very precious. For that reason, it's so important not to take it or those you love and care about for granted because one day any one of them could be gone. It's not a question of if; it's a question of when (for all of us).

In addition to working on my book, trying to keep up with all the e-mails, going through treatments, recuperating from seizures, and fighting this cancer, I have also decided to make my final arrangements in the chance that I may pass on to heaven unexpectedly. It will be on my mind until I get it done. So, in order to have some peace about the issue, I am going to have to facilitate this immediately. Then I will have the reassurance that certain decisions are not left for those who remain behind after I'm gone. Of course, I hope and pray I can make it to at least eighty. That's what Michael and I have agreed to, anyway.

Because my husband accidently hit two deer while driving to work recently, our headlight is out. Therefore, all of our driving has to take place during the day to avoid getting a ticket. However, our plan to get back home before dark was derailed due to the fact we had to spend over three hours waiting at the pharmacy in Encinitas, trying to get the thalidomide prescription filled.

Finally, after a lot of hassle and red tape, they got it ready for us, but not before first ringing it up on our card without telling us what the charge was. The preposterous price turned out to be $5,300 for only a twenty-eight-day cycle. Considering everything, we just don't happen to have that in our back pockets. You would think they would have had the intelligence and the courtesy to mention that little detail before they rung us up.

The fact is, as previously mentioned, we paid close to $500 a month for health insurance to cover that. The consequence was that we were forced to pay for another room at the Holiday Inn that night while we waited for the twenty-four-to-forty-eight-hour turnaround to get the Thalidomide at the discounted price. And, of course, the broken headlights are keeping us here anyway.

Tomorrow, I will get my PET scan results from Dr. McClay. The doctor at Scripts looked at my MRI scans and concluded that my brain hemorrhages/seizures were not from his Gamma Knife procedures. He suspects that they were from a previous procedure at USC—either from that or a new lesion. We hope and pray it is not the former.

We arrived safely home in Pahrump by around 5:00 p.m. the next evening, thankfully before the sunset. Amanda decided to stay at home by herself that night instead of going to her dad's, as she usually did while I was working. She said it just felt too good to be back home in her own bed. And, of course, there were the "boys," which we both missed when we were gone.

Although the doctors didn't want Amanda to be left unsupervised, she had her dad's number on speed dial if she started to remotely feel like she did prior to having the seizures and brain aneurisms. And she checked in with both her dad and me throughout the night to let us know she was okay. After the holidays, Michelle, a good friend of Amanda's, had planned to come and stay with us to help with our situation.

At this point my wife had to schedule a once-a-week infusion with the chemo Taxotere in addition to her daily amino acid infusions, Monday through Friday. And while she got a break from the infusions on the weekends, she had to take over thirty pills just to make up for their two-day absence.

The next day we received her PET scan results, which were bitter sweet. We were both expecting that her lung tumors had increased dramatically in size since she had so many new sub-q lesions popping up all over her body of late, but Dr. McClay was pleasantly surprised to report that those tumors had only increased a very small amount since they were last measured in October. Frankly, he was expecting a much more discouraging report.

Amanda started taking the Temodar again that night—120 mg each evening for six weeks. The doctor felt that this should help to keep any new brain mets away until she was healthy enough to try the immunotherapy injections again. He also stressed that he wanted her to keep up with the nutritional immunotherapy that she was getting from Dr. Royal in Vegas.

In Amanda's Words...

Just a quick note to reiterate that just because I am working on making my final arrangements at thirty-one years old does not mean I am giving up on this fight in the slightest. In fact, for me, getting things worked out ahead of time will give me more strength to focus on healing, enjoying life and getting better that much sooner. I will have less stress once I have worked out all the decisions, and I believe it will give me that much more focus and clarity to be able to heal from this absolutely horrific disease.

Today I worked on our house, cleaning and unpacking from our trip to San Diego. I ripped up some carpet from my master closet and sorted through much of the clutter that has accumulated since we moved in last year. Ironically, this whole experience has also made me value clutter more than I ever did. I am going through everything, which will take some time, but weeding out all of the non-necessary stuff will be beneficial for us both in the long run. If I haven't used it in a year, I probably won't again and therefore will put it in the yard sale pile off the back porch. This pile is quickly growing, so we just might be able to get rid of some stuff and make some funds to help with our expenses while doing it.

I currently have some really sore tumor spots around the areas that have not been injected. I am hoping and praying that my immune system, although severely compromised, is fighting some of these tumors off. I feel a little more reassured now that I'm back on Temodar for the brain mets. Hopefully it will stop any new ones from forming anytime soon.

I apologize in advance if it takes a while for me to respond to your e-mails. Some take longer than others, especially with us being out of town and doing treatments every day. Please be patient, and in time, one of us will get back to you.

There is so much new information to report, but it will have to wait until I get some time this weekend to give all the details. I'll try to give another update real soon. Just wanted you to know that I/we are okay and in pretty high spirits. I've been having e-mail and computer issues lately, which have taken up a lot of my time. Plus I've been in Vegas every day getting the infusions, which take a couple hours each, and one day a week, I am getting two (one for chemo and the other for the immunotherapy amino acids). I will work on writing up all the details when I'm able. In the meantime, know that we are all right and keeping busy as ever.

A Hammer to Her Head;
A Knife to my Heart

Shortly before Christmas, Amanda began suffering from an intense migraine headache, so I stayed home with her all day, as we debated whether or not to go to the emergency room. Although it's difficult to imagine, things were becoming increasingly *more* challenging for her. Between the effects of all the new chemo in combination with her still swollen brain, just holding any kind of thought really took major effort. She also was experiencing severe tightness through her jaw and temple areas.

Most of the day was spent simply striving to decrease Amanda's pain through any means possible. In addition, she had recently been forced to increase her dose of Dexameth to accommodate the extra swelling. Dr. McClay wanted to wean her off of that particular drug, as it lowers the immune system, but as long as the chronic pounding in her head continued, she had no other choice but to take it. It also caused significant swelling in her face, which only compounded the intense discomfort in her jaw and temples. Nevertheless, it did help ease the brain swelling, which was so important, and when she took a full dose of Dexameth, she was able to keep that at least somewhat at bay. It's amazing how incapacitated one becomes when the brain swells. The simplest thought overwhelmed her, and she had a great deal of difficulty processing the most basic information. She would forget what she was doing at any given point in time and got confused and frustrated (understandably) very easily. Just getting dressed, updating the website, or answering normal e-mails—things she once did so routinely—proved to be a monumental challenge. She noticed that her hand/eye coordination was also off, as whenever she tried to reach for something, inevitably the item was several inches away from her outstretched hand. The after effects of the seizures and brain hemorrhage she had experienced a few weeks earlier definitely had a huge impact on her ability to function. However, as was the hallmark of my precious wife, she continued to try her best to keep calm and learn more about what was happening to her.

In Amanda's Words...

I have another interesting day for us today. There is so much to say, but it's too late right now for all the details. I will update more in the morning. Basically, the two tumors in my brain have gotten bigger to where I have lost some of my vision and cognitive responses. The tumors are both now about the size of golf balls and causing pressure all the time. Wishing you a very Merry Christmas.

Although I did my best to deny it, our developing reality was extremely bleak. Amanda had to be re-hospitalized, and when I entered her room, I leaned over, and we both cried and repeated our love for each other.

But, of course, I felt I had to pull myself together, as I couldn't bear to increase her emotional discomfort on top of everything else. Amanda's dad; his wife, Vickie; Kristi; Craig; and my twin brother, Ron, all showed up that evening. When Kristi approached her bedside, Amanda immediately held her so tightly I thought she was never going to let go. Tears started falling from Kristi's eyes as she embraced her sister. Amanda said, "Kristi, I love you so much. Forgive me for any of the bad things in the—"

Kristi stopped her right there and said, "I'm sorry too, but the past is the past. We have a future to get on with. I love you." It was the most perfect demonstration of sisterly adoration I have ever witnessed.

Next, Ron came up to the bed at Amanda's request. She said to him, "I'm so sorry for the fighting we did," and Ron said the very same thing back to her. Then she said something that all who watched the scene unfold will never forget: "Water under the bridge." Tears started falling from Ron's eyes as he hugged her. While she was visiting with the family, I walked over to the nurses' station and talked with Dr. Sief. He told me that things weren't good. There was a golf-ball-size tumor in her left occipital lobe, one in her right occipital lobe, and one near her cerebellum near the brain stem. The prognosis was, in a word, bad—something I'd been told more times than I cared to count. He said that it was mandatory to do a brain surgery right away. I remember having to wait for hours to get an ambulance to transport us, but we were finally taken to Sunrise Hospital, the best facility in the area for such a delicate operation. It was four hours later than it should have been, and I know Amanda was very upset about it, but we finally arrived at the hospital. Luckily, Amanda was able to get a little sleep.

Our Fairytale Turns Grim

In Amanda's Words...

Here is hoping you all had the most wonderful holidays with your families and friends. I myself have been spending some of the best quality time ever with mine, and it's been really good for my heart. There have been lots of major changes happening lately. We are currently faced with some serious decisions and can use all the positive prayers and good thoughts you can spare during this time. We discovered that I have three tumors in my brain now, one that needs to be operated on immediately. I have surgery scheduled for this Friday, the 30th, at 7:30 a.m. I'd be lying if I said I wasn't scared. Brain surgery is a pretty major thing to undergo. However, it has become necessary at this juncture. I have the love and support of my family and friends and complete faith in God, so I am not worried. I know things will be just fine no matter what the outcome. I do want to take a moment and thank each of you for all of the continued love, support, and concern you've shown to Michael and me through this battle we've been waging for the past year. It's so helped to keep us both strong, and it's extremely important that you know how much it means to us.

Amanda's Mother Remembers...

So much has gone on since my last letter in November, but I will try to cover the basics. Many of you check Mandy's website for news, but she hasn't been able to write many updates as of late, as she has had an increasingly difficult time recovering from the seizures in November.

At first it seemed the prescribed steroid (Dexameth) was controlling the swelling from the ruptured tumor, but she needed ever increasing doses to keep the headaches at bay. She also started to notice a big change in her vision and hand-eye coordination in addition to an overall fuzzy, foggy feeling where she just couldn't think clearly.

December 18th, Michael was playing with ShaNaNa at the Sun Coast, and since all the family was in town, she and Michael arranged for us to attend the show. We had a wonderful time!

December 19th, her sister, Kristi, was graduating college, and Mandy very much wanted to be in attendance. Although she hadn't been out of bed for more than a few hours at a time since the seizures, Mandy rose to the occasion and attended the ShaNaNa concert. In addition, the next day, she attended Kristi's graduation ceremony, celebration dinner, and party afterward. Although she had some difficulties, her headaches were much less frequent and severe and she had a great time.

December 20th, the headaches and fuzzy thinking returned with a vengeance. We thought it was caused by all the activity of the past few days, and she needed more rest to recuperate.

Over the holidays she rested but just didn't bounce back as hoped. Each day required more and more Dexameth to keep the headaches away. Her thinking had become quite muddled, and it was very frustrating for her.

Trying to reach doctors during the holidays is very difficult. However, she did meet with Dr. Michael's assistant (from Las Vegas Comprehensive Cancer Center) who ordered an MRI.

Monday (December 28th), Mandy was feeling much worse. Her thinking was visibly compromised, and she was feeling lightheaded with hazy vision. Michael called to tell me he was bringing her into emergency. I called Dr. Sief (neurosurgeon who treated her when she had the hemorrhage), who arranged to have her admitted to Sunrise Hospital. Additional scans showed three tumors (two we knew about in the occipital lobe and one new one).

Mandy's team of doctors (a neurosurgeon, radiologist, and her two oncologists) agreed she would require surgery to remove this new, particularly fast-growing tumor located in a very sensitive area in her brain. Although it is in the outermost region, the rapid growth and swelling is putting immense and dangerous pressure on her central nerve trunk, which controls vital body function (heart, breathing, etc.). Mandy will have surgery early Friday morning, and I'll be flying in tomorrow. I plan on staying a week or two to help with Mandy's recovery and treatments.

Needless to say, Mandy hoped to avoid surgery if at all possible, but sadly, any other method of treating this tumor (radiation, etc.) would likely increase the swelling, which is already at a dangerous level. The surgery is expected to be about one hour long, followed by about five to eight days of recuperation. Once the tumor is removed, the swelling should subside and most—if not all—of the headaches and other symptoms should be relieved. They will not be surgically removing the other two tumors but instead plan to treat them with radiation after she recovers from the surgery.

I wish I could report that the combined surgery and radiation would "cure" her melanoma, but it won't. What it will do is rid her of the brain tumors (causing the headaches, etc.) and give her additional time. Mandy still is fighting and unwilling to accept defeat. She plans to resume her chemotherapy and is in hopes of adding Anvirzel (a very new treatment drug derived from Oleander) to her regimen.

Please keep your prayers and well wishes coming.

It was right before the brain surgery; I believe two days prior. We were in her room at the hospital, and her mom, dad, and sister were all there. We had a nice visit with them—as pleasant as could be expected. Anyway, there was a lot of loving going on, and that was wonderful to see. (I knew in my heart how important this time was for them as a family). When the hugs and kisses were over and everyone left, I had some quiet time with Amanda. We talked about our house and our cats. She always wanted them near her. After a few hours of talking and resting, she was feeling hungry. Because I didn't want her to have hospital food, I gave her a big kiss and said I'd be right back. I drove down Eastern going south and turned into a parking lot on Flamingo. I was in a search for sushi, one of Amanda's favorite foods. Finally, I found a place. I walked in and said to the chef, "I want one order of everything!"

The guy looked at me and said, "Excuse me, you want what?"

I said, "You heard me right."

After briefly explaining why I ordered that way, he nodded his head with respect and condolence and said, "Give me forty-five minutes." I then went to my friend

Dennis's house, which was nearby. I needed to just cry my head off—the stress I was feeling was unbelievable! Then I would remember that it was Amanda, not me, who was sitting in a hospital bed, and my stress disappeared. I went back to the sushi place, and the chef had thirteen bags full of the stuff. The bill was over $500. He gave it to me for $300.

I had enough sushi to feed a football team! As I entered her room with the bags and bags of food, Amanda looked up at me as if Santa Claus had just dropped down the chimney! After opening up all of the boxes, it looked like sushi had rained down from the ceiling.

Amanda just glanced up at me and said, "Please pass me the wasabi, honey." She was so awesome! We gobbled down the food like there was no tomorrow, which at that point, we didn't know if there would be for us. Nonetheless, it was a feast fit for royalty, and Amanda gleefully presided over the whole occasion, feeding every nurse and orderly on duty in the process! In spite of the dire situation looming on the horizon, I must say, it was one of the best times we ever spent together, a memory forever emblazoned in my heart and mind.

Profile in Courage

In Amanda's Words…

So much has been going on as of late, where to begin? Let me first start by saying that we hope your New Year has started off and continues to be a wonderful beginning. It has been for us a beginning of renewed hope and blessing of more time in this life.

Although I was barely able to even sit up, I thankfully had the strength to make it to see my sister graduate from college and attend her dinner and party afterward. However, as the night progressed, I kept feeling more and more pressure in my head, and finally, it just got to be too much.

On the morning of December 30th, I went through a brain surgery to remove a tumor in my left occipital lobe. The tumor was the size of a golf ball and had grown twice its size since the end of October 2005. Michael is helping me recall all the details because I don't remember much, just bits and pieces of the whole experience. There is another almond-size tumor in my right occipital lobe and one more in my cerebellum.

Tomorrow morning, January 6th, I will undergo my first brain radiation treatment.

We are just going to do low doses, twelve to fifteen times. Each treatment takes about ten to fifteen minutes. I'm not sure about the side effects from radiation on the brain. However, I am a pro when it comes to everywhere else, so I know something of what to expect. Out of all the treatments that I have had to endure, the radiation seems to be the easiest and most tolerable one. The downfall with this brain radiation is that it is a claustrophobic feeling where they have my whole head restrained. I have to lie on the area where I had the incision from the surgery for about fifteen minutes each session, definitely a no-fun zone. However, the radiation seems to be working on my sacral spinal canal tumor, so I have high hopes for this next fight against this melanoma cancer.

Although the immunotherapy is starting to work now too, it can be pretty grueling. Many of the injected spots are very hard, and some are starting to come through my skin. They are hideous and sore right now. It makes it very difficult to find a comfortable spot to just be in, but I manage. As soon as each of these comes through the skin and out, that means there's one less tumor my body has to try to fight off. That is a good thing!

My stomach has been distended real badly for the past five days or so. I think it is mostly from being in the hospital and continuing to be on all the meds. I've tried all kinds of things for it, but it still hasn't gone down yet. I might have to look into getting all the extra fluid drained; I'm not sure. God bless everyone for your prayers. They have helped me through all of this more than you'll ever know.

Soon after the brain operation, we were momentarily encouraged. Amanda was able to see better. Whereas before, when I would put my hand up, she wouldn't be able to see it; now she could. Her writing was also corrected, which was especially satisfying to her.

A very short time later, my mother was getting married in Hawaii. Because my entire family was going to be there, they really wanted us to join them in the celebration. Amanda and I talked about it and decided we'd attempt the trip—a miracle considering what she'd gone through literally just days earlier. And although it had been her fondest desire to take me where she had grown up in Grass Valley, California, she sacrificed that dream so I could be at my mother's wedding. She was *so* unreal.

We still had a very nice time during this brief reprieve, as Amanda's sister, Kristi, flew in for the event, as well. I remember Amanda at the Kona Airport. Kristi had just gotten off the plane, and Amanda hid from Kristi as she went to get her luggage. Moments later, she snuck up and tapped Kristi on the shoulder. They both screamed like little schoolgirls and hugged each other for what seemed to be at least five minutes. Amanda put the traditional lei on Kristi and welcomed her to Hawaii.

I wanted to do something extra special for my wife while we were there, and my mother told us about a cove in the area called Kahaluu Beach, which is world renowned for snorkeling. As I figured, it was the "softest" experience she could have (at least the one with the most minimal impact to her body), we agreed to give it a try; in fact, Amanda was *adamant* that we must. So, I purchased a wet suit that fit her snugly and, although she experienced a certain amount of pain in putting it on, snorkeling was something she had always wanted to try, and we both knew this was going to be her last opportunity to dive in.

The unique thing about this location was that you didn't need a boat to see the most amazing fish; in fact, you could just wade in. And while it was rocky going in some areas, Amanda was absolutely determined to do it herself…completely unassisted. In fact, she actually got annoyed when several people offered to help. For even at this point, my wife had a way of getting her point across in the most diplomatic yet firmest of manners. "Leave me alone, I've got it!" she bellowed. This was her show, and it was a one-woman performance.

With Kristi bidding us adieu from the shore, I followed meekly behind. Once we were in deep enough to swim, I held her hand as we watched, with great fascination, God's undersea extravaganza unfold. My brother, Ron, and niece, Natasha, had preceded us into the ocean, and she decided to provide the big bang to the outing with a watery fireworks display. As such, she opened up a bag of the peas that are used as "catnip" for tropical fish. Although only a small handful is usually required to get their attention, this trip had nothing to do with the status quo. Natasha threw the whole bag out and sat back, watching for the absolute feeding frenzy that was about to occur. Within seconds, hundreds of tropical fish were surrounding Amanda, gobbling up the smorgasbord that had just been laid out at their fishy, little feet. Amanda felt like Ariel, the Disney mermaid princess, holding court at the table's head. What a panorama unfolded, as the rainbow of flutters seemed to have been choreographed to dance in perfect synchronization around her. Amanda was so overcome with joy, we could actually hear her giggling in the underwater world in which we were immersed. A truly glorious day!

The next morning, while Amanda, Kristi, and I were having breakfast near the breathtakingly beautiful shoreline, we noticed some little birds flying around the tables, hoping to get some scraps of food. Amanda threw out some pieces of her toast and giggled as the birds tried to get the bread. After each successful grab, another bird would steal it only seconds later. I even laughed at this and was especially thrilled by the subsequent event. For about halfway through our meal, we saw some people pointing out at the ocean. All of a sudden, a huge whale jumped almost completely out of the water! It was a dazzling display of God's omnipresence and most certainly a sight to remember.

In retrospect, having Kristi there was so important, as she provided Amanda with her side of the family. At such a critical time, she stepped up to the plate and became the best sister anyone could wish for.

Don't Cry Out Loud

In Amanda's bathroom there were big mirrors, and one day as I was helping her out of the bath, she caught a glimpse of her completely tumor-ridden body in all of its horror. She turned to me with the most crest-fallen expression I have ever seen and shrieked, "Michael, they are all over me!" Tears started to fall, and not just hers. I ran to her and held her as we cried together.

In Amanda's Words...

So much to say, so little energy to say it all. The radiation treatments have made my body want to sleep all the time. In fact, at midday my eyes often close automatically, and I can't reopen them, but I had been warned that sleepiness and hair loss were two of the biggest side effects of radiation. Also, I no longer can use my stomach muscles for anything like lifting myself up. The radiologist said it was the body's way of repairing itself after good cells were killed off during the treatment.

Finally, yesterday was the first day I didn't have to get any more radiation on my abdomen, which was such a relief, though I continue to receive the treatments on my brain.

My stomach is so sore it feels as though I've been punched about a thousand times. Partly it's the radiation; partly it's the immunotherapy starting to work as the numerous tumors come out all over my back, neck, and other body parts. What really concerns me the most are all the new sub-q tumors that have come up all over my head. I've spent the majority of my time back from Hawaii sleeping and recuperating. Luckily for me, we will visit again very soon, as my husband is performing with ShaNaNa, so we can stay at the Hilton Waikoloa Hotel. I hope we can accomplish all we had wanted to last time since we had to leave earlier than we wanted to.

I took my pain journal off this site because I thought it was a little monotonous to write about it all in two different places—too much work. But when I actually stopped writing in that journal, I stopped writing about my pain almost entirely.

However, as those closest to me have pointed out, this journey has been more difficult than has been conveyed on the site. It is certainly not as "easy" as it appears. In fact, it is the hardest thing that either Michael or I have ever had to endure. I left some parts out because it seemed enough to feel my pain, much less write about, too.

It's true that writing about it kind of squashes any kind of denial I may have had about my personal reality, but that was not the main reason. I really didn't want to be the cause of anyone else's worry or sorrow. I have the personality that is the type where, if another person is hurt, I empathize to the point I can sometimes actually physically feel their pain or feelings. That pain is elevated when I know I am, in some way, the cause. I have experienced this type of empathy since I was a child. The fact is I want so much for my story to be about a miracle, a life rescued from cancer. That is my prayer.

We drive to see Dr. McClay first thing tomorrow and then back to Vegas for more brain radiation. May peace and love be with you all.

PS - And I thought having major back surgery was bad! Ha!

It was Super Bowl Sunday, and Amanda was experiencing a tremendous amount of pain. Although she really couldn't eat, I was trying my best to feed her. However, as soon as she got it down, her stomach pain increased. We left for Encinitas at 3:00 a.m. and arrived at the doctor's office five hours later. I was acutely aware that time was of the essence and something had to be done for her immediately, as her breathing was becoming compromised as well.

I had made the back seat as comfortable as possible for my wife, but she was still feeling every little bump in the road. At this stage of the disease, it was so very painful that just seeing a bump ahead was almost enough to send Amanda screaming through the roof.

Amanda had started her new treatment that afternoon: a very long infusion, taking almost five hours. We also learned during the visit that she has a tumor the size of an egg located right in the middle of her chest. I prayed with all my heart that, by some miracle, the new treatment would work, but in my gut I knew the odds were against her.

In Amanda's Words...

Michael has been updating the website for me sometimes when I am too weak or tired, which I appreciate so much. My poor, darling husband, like he doesn't already have enough on his plate.

This daily radiation has made things really difficult for us in more ways than one. It makes me want to sleep, and that's about it. My husband has to drive me into Vegas every day for treatment, drive right back, and then turn around and make the 120-mile, round-trip journey again for work almost every night. Today the car was broken, so we actually got a day at home. What a treat that was!

I haven't been able to eat hardly at all lately. Although I'm trying to maintain my weight, I have to literally force-feed myself. The past five days, I've also gotten sick every time I've tried to put anything in my stomach. So now, with the help of antinausea meds I am slowly getting my appetite back. Tumors have started to come up all over, many sub-qs. These were older ones that were injected—the two on my face, the two on my neck, and the two on my upper shoulder, which are huge and look somewhat like eyeballs. I also have a very low red blood cell count, and they said I would need a blood transfusion. I did receive a shot of Arinesp, so hopefully that will bring it up again. We start on new medication soon, hoping that will be our answer.

We did receive some good news recently— the tumor that was radiated in my abdomen has decreased in size from an eight to a 5.5!

I'm in a lot of pain lately with these things coming up all over my body. When I find a comfortable position, I usually will stay for a while.

Michael helps me out of the car and with walking when we go get radiation treatment in Vegas or elsewhere. I just finished the videos I wanted to make for my family, in case I should pass. What a weight lifted now that those are done! They were, however, very emotionally draining to do.

Circle of Life

Going to the radiologist's was so very uncomfortable for Amanda. We would walk down a long hallway and into another room—kind of like a maze—which housed a very large machine that would circle around her body. That was the easy part. Getting Amanda into a comfortable position was the supreme challenge. First they fit her into her body and scalp molds and then they laid her down and strapped the molds onto the table very snugly. They do this so the radiation is centered where they need it, and so her body wouldn't move. And although this worked for a few times, as the tumors grew, the pain of having them smashed when she was placed on the table was unbearable, causing tears to stream down her face.

While the doctor tried to put soft pillows under her for cushioning, it didn't matter after a certain point. I could blow air on the tumors, and they would hurt her.

In Amanda's Words...

It's the last week of February and we are *blessed* to once again be in beautiful Kona, Hawaii where Michael is playing with ShaNaNa. Unfortunately, my energy level is severely lacking. All I want to do is sleep, but then I can very rarely find a comfortable position due to the massive amounts of tumors that are present. Michael is trying to set up a blood transfusion immediately since my red counts are so dangerously low.

Things are tough right now, and I am in a lot of pain. My meds have been increased due to the agony I'm experiencing at the tumor sites. I'm hoping and praying that this transfusion will give me the life force I need.

While in our hotel room, Amanda was experiencing a great deal of pain, so I gave her some morphine pills. However, fearing that I might overdose her, I wasn't giving her enough to manage the intense discomfort. I felt so badly that she had to suffer because of that.

God only knows how, but she did muster the intestinal fortitude to come and see me perform with Sha Na Na that night. But because there were no tables available in the room, she grabbed my sister, Shari, and took her around the corner to sit and listen. As I was playing "In the Still of the Night" on stage, Amanda - assured I couldn't overhear - took the opportunity to at last articulate to Shari, the person in whom she had ultimately chosen to confide, the most poignant and reluctant realization of her life: she wasn't going to make it. As she poured her heart out to my sister, they spoke of love, loss, and life; as well as of her profound sadness and regret at not being able to give me the child we both had longed for. Most importantly, however, it finally gave Amanda the chance to reveal to someone close her ultimate truth. As they hugged and sobbed, my sister reiterated to my wife how very deeply she was loved and asked, that as a sign of her eternalness, Amanda somehow divinely arrange to place a white rose where she'd least expect to find one. With that, came the final note of what we had always considered to be "our" song. It was also the last time Amanda was ever to hear me sing.

Later on that day, she was not doing well at all. I took her to the hospital where she needed a blood transfusion and, fortunately, they gave her Dilaudid, a painkiller, which seemed to work.

I remember her saying, "This stuff works great. I don't feel any pain!" But her words made me cry. It had been too long for her to be in such constant agony.

The next morning she was strong enough to accompany me to church. It was a wonderful service, and there were so many people praying for Amanda. It is still extremely emotional for me to replay those heart-breaking memories.

In Amanda's Words...

We decided to cut our Hawaii trip short by a couple of days, as I was in too much pain to do anything but stay in bed. It was nice to see Mike perform with ShaNaNa again, though. He impressed his wife, as always, and of course the crowd and the band as well.

When we returned home, we had the hospice come over to our house, even though I am still fighting. They signed me up and changed my meds to 45 mg of long-acting morphine, which seems to help a lot more than the Hydrocodone did.

I didn't want to go on hospice originally, but I think it's now the best solution to my current health state. I hope their services will alleviate some of Michael's stress as well.

We flew down to Dr. McClay's and had a meeting with him in addition to getting another infusion of the two chemotherapies. His opinion was that if I am not able to get these things under control, my prognosis would be three to six months.

He wants us to start Velcade too, which involves going to San Diego twice a week for the injections. These injections are going to run $600 each. We are thinking of either having to refinance our house or, hopefully, we can put on a benefit that might be able to cover it.

Thirty Days

After her visit with the doctor, I left Amanda with our friends, Paul and Roberta, and maneuvered my way back to his office. Entering a little abruptly, I seemed to startle him for just a second. Then he turned to me and, in a very soft voice with great depth of feeling, said, "Oh, hello, Michael. What can I do for you?"

Knowing what this probably meant, I became very scared. Choking down the tears, I asked him, "What are our chances?"

He looked at me, his eyes laden with sadness, and solemnly replied, "Michael, I give her 0 percent chance of getting rid of this…and I give a 10 to 15 percent chance of stopping it momentarily."

The lump in my throat seemed to almost pop out of my mouth as my mind raced for some port on which to anchor my thoughts. I just kept repeating, "Oh my *God*…Dr. McClay was the best we could find! What do I do?" As I shook his hand, I instinctively knew it was my final exchange with a man I had come to care about, respect, and, most of all, rely upon like no other.

But I was absolutely resolute about not telling Amanda his prognosis. I needed to keep her hopes alive at all costs. I loved her so very much, and I found myself losing it more and more as I watched her slip further and further away every day. Anyone who knows me well will tell you that I can literally sob at the drop of a hat. In fact, if I had fully allowed myself to react to what was happening, I would have been crying twenty-three hours a day.

My wife was trying to sleep, but it was extremely difficult for her. There were so many tumors at this point there was simply no escape from the havoc they were wrecking on her largely defenseless little body. Whether she was sitting or lying down, it didn't matter! The only time she wasn't feeling complete excruciation was when she was sleeping. Amanda was then up to three Loritab pills and a morphine pill per pain session. And while I struggled to maintain an iota of flickering hope, I feared Amanda was losing the war with this murderous foe. I vividly remember just trying to kiss her and my nose hitting a tumor underneath her left eye. From that time on, I could only kiss her on one side of her face.

A few days later, Amanda started seeing spots on the bedroom wall. Naturally, they were for her eyes only, but nonetheless, I asked her to point them out in a feeble attempt to try and comprehend what she was going through. She reached out and pointed, then quickly pointed again and again. They were all around her, about a foot away. She said they were different colors, and that they looked kind of "pretty."

In my own frantic state of mind, I knew what this meant, and it wasn't good. At the same time, her handwriting started to change. When she began to write something, her hand would slide down before the end of her sentence. She could not keep her writing level on the paper.

This really bothered her, as she prided herself on her penmanship and excellent grammar, and was extremely scary for both of us.

Unfortunately, I still had to make a living; so it was off to another night on the old bandstand. I told Amanda that I would do the show and come right back...and I did. Upon my arrival, as always, I immediately rushed to her side. But when I touched her, she was absolutely drenched in sweat. After I got her up and dried her off, we stood next to the window, embracing as we gazed out at a world that had once held such promise for us. Before going back to bed, I helped her into some dry pajamas and, placing a towel over the side on which she'd been sleeping, led her around to the other one. Ever the lady even in the direst of circumstances, she actually thanked me for taking the wet side!

Emotionally, I felt tremendous pain in being the husband of a woman who was fighting for her life. I also felt enormous pride and joy as the husband of a woman who simply refused to accept defeat.

By then, even the simple act of getting out of bed exhausted Amanda, so I tucked her in and then assumed my treasured position next to her. She turned to her left side, and I wrapped my body, as gently as I could, around hers. Finally, I heard a weak but contented sigh eek out of her, as she drifted off. After she was asleep, I started to pray. I think I said something like, "I'll make a deal with you, God..." I'm sure you get the picture. I had to wipe my tears before they landed on Amanda's arm. I didn't want to wake her up.

Our last trip to see Dr. Sharda was heart wrenching. I needed to use a wheelchair to get Amanda around. There was a tumor the size of a grapefruit in her bowel area that they needed to radiate ASAP. Amanda was standing up while they got little foam balls so that she might be able to lie down. I heard her scream with pain as Dr. Sharda accidentally hit a tumor on her back. As she wept in agony, I could see Dr. Sharda lower his head. He was behind Amanda so she couldn't see him, but I noticed how devastated he was for accidentally hurting her. I got the feeling that if he could have wept…he would have too.

By March, Amanda required an oxygen tank at home. Strangely, when I heard it hum, I derived a small comfort in the knowledge that at least she was getting good air. By then, comforts were few and far between. Her pain meds had been increased to 60 mgs both morning and night, and she still was taking the liquid morphine for breakthrough pain. Around that time she told me that there were new tumors in her jaw and throat. What could I say other than, "I love you?" It was all I knew.

Benefit of the Doubt

We were planning to have another fund-raiser for Amanda the following Wednesday night at the Forty Deuce. Of course over the months and months of treatment, the bills we had accumulated were through the roof and continually rising, but I didn't care. There was no cost too high for Amanda's life and my pat phrase was, "Just put it on my tab." Nevertheless, we had hoped we could defray at least a tiny portion of the expenses through this event.

Although she was going to try and be there, and I encouraged her to do so if she felt strong enough, it didn't really matter in the big picture. All that counted was that we were trying our hardest to make things as nice as humanly possible for her. That morning she had managed to gift me with one of her trademark smiles; the most beautiful I had ever seen, especially because it took such effort on her part to provide.

While Amanda looked a little better the next a.m., she still wasn't able to eat. But regardless of the fact that I felt as though I was falling into a bottomless pit, I knew I'd never again experience the pure love we shared and relished every second of our togetherness. It still fills my heart with pride and joy to this day whenever I think of her undying devotion and utter grace under the most extraordinary pressure imaginable—a consummate class act.

Ultimately, Amanda wasn't well enough to attend the event in her honor, but nonetheless, Connie helped her get dressed in the beautiful turquoise-blue blouse and crème-colored pants she had bought her especially for the occasion. As I listened to my dear friend Michael Grimm perform with his band, I called Amanda on my cell so she could hear him, too. As soon as he finished one of his songs, I put the wireless microphone up to the phone so she could say something to the crowd. She told them how she wished she could have been there and thanked them so much for all of their support. "Have a drink for me!" she chirped as merrily as a young woman on the precipice of the great unknown could sound.

As soon as she was finished, the cheering and applause from the crowd was deafening, with nary a dry eye in the house. I remember Michael lowered his head and, hugging me with all of his might, whispered, "I love you, man," as his tears pressed against my cheek. In spite of the unthinkable hardship that was now her life, my gutsy wife once again rallied to the fore. I couldn't have been prouder of or more humbled by anyone.

From behind the scenes, Connie reported:
The night of the benefit, Mandy was not feeling well at all. She so wanted to be there, pushing herself beyond all limits to make it. But the one-hour drive each way plus an hour or so at the benefit was more than she had the strength to endure. After some discussion, we decided that Michael would go, and if Mandy

felt stronger, I would drive her in to attend. As the evening wore on, it became apparent she just didn't have the stamina to make the trip. Therefore we compromised, coming up with the idea of Michael calling on his cell phone and holding it to the mike, allowing her to speak directly the audience.

Mandy was not only feeling weak but also was having some trouble concentrating. She began to get nervous about how to best to convey her thanks to everyone. It would have been easier face-to-face, but over the phone, she thought it just felt so formal. She decided to jot down what she planned to say to be sure she didn't forget anything. I arranged the pillows so she could sit comfortably and found a tablet on which she could write. She thought for a little bit and began. After she had written one line, she stopped and stared at the notepad. I thought she was thinking of what to say next, but then she glanced up with an expression of terror. My heart instantly raced. Then calmly, she said, "Mom, look how small my writing is. It feels like I'm writing normally, but the letters are so tiny." Indeed, while her handwriting (which was always large and round), looked the same; it was now in miniature form, not even taking up a quarter of the space on the page. She became frantic as she remembered the last time that this had happened was just prior to the seizures and was terrified she was going to start seizing again. Naturally, I neither knew the answer to her question nor how to reply to it. Her fear cut through me, and I was desperate to alleviate it and somehow make it right. I simply had no clue as to how to accomplish this.

I don't think I gave her any answer, but rather remember saying something like, "Well, maybe it's better you don't write it all out anyway. Then it won't sound like you are reading a script. Just say what comes to your mind. I know you'll do just fine." Moments later, Michael called, and I handed her the phone. Mandy began to speak without any hesitation or sign of nervousness. She spoke from her heart, thanking family and friends for their support and even ending with a little joke. She did wonderfully.

After the call she was relaxed and seemed to be feeling a little better. We talked for a while, and then she took a snooze while she waited for Michael to come home and tell her all about the evening.

We had a wonderful turnout and collected enough money to pay for six more weeks of Amanda's treatment. My gratitude for this absolutely amazing outpouring of love was truly beyond words.

Last Call

By now, the chemo wasn't working like her doctor would have liked, so we scheduled a blood test close to home before we drove down for her next round the following Tuesday. It was agreed that Anvirzel was her best (and possibly only) shot, but as we were living on borrowed time and the drug takes at least three months to become effective, her chances were pretty slim that it could actually be of any help.

It was the first week of April 2006, and since we didn't have money to fly, we drove to Dr. Steenblock's clinic in Orange County. As a last ditch effort, we were going to explore stem cell research. In spite of the fact that Amanda's condition was worsening by the day, we nevertheless, had to keep on keeping on. When we got there and sat down with Dr. Steenblock, his bedside manner proved, once again, absolutely atrocious. Amanda did not like it one bit. But in spite of this fact, I did appreciate his willingness to provide her with a glimmer of hope when we had exhausted every other flicker and flame.

During the course of our conversation, Amanda had to go to the bathroom, and as soon as she got out the door, the doctor looked at me and said, "Stem cell research takes about a month to take. She doesn't have a month."

With those words, I felt as though my heart was going to stop beating. Of course, it wasn't as though every other doctor hadn't arrived at a similar conclusion, but the thought of her actual demise wasn't something—even then—I could allow my mind to accept.

Because I only had a couple of minutes before Amanda would come back to join us, I quickly asked the doctor to please not relay what he had told me to my wife. She had already had the doom and gloom prognosis and possessed a greater reality of her true condition than perhaps anyone else—medical miracle workers included. With all of my might, I tried to maintain her hope, as it was all she had left. I simply couldn't take that away from her, too.

Antabuse pills, a hyperbaric chamber, and vitamin C drips—the former of which I administered to her at home—were the only treatment options we were left with; but at least they were *something*.

We had just passed Victorville on our drive back home when Amanda indicated with her hand movement that she wanted me to go around a truck that was in front of us. The next thing I knew, we were stuck in a horrific, bumper-to-bumper traffic jam due to roadwork. It was nighttime and pouring rain, but Amanda said she had to go to the bathroom. Knowing she would never make it to the next off ramp and stuck in the middle of the desert in the pouring rain, I looked up to the sky and prayed for the Lord's help. Miraculously, not a minute later, a huge tree—the only one I'd seen in over a hundred miles – seemed to appear out of nowhere on the right hand side of the road. I pulled over and, as gently as I could, helped her out of the car before holding her under the arms so she could relieve herself in "private."

I want to emphasize how thankful I was to God for putting that tree there for Amanda to relieve herself. I almost started to cry with happiness that He heard my prayer and immediately responded with His loving care.

As we continued our drive, she suddenly looked over at me and said, "Michael...what if the worst happens?" Turning my head to the left in a futile attempt to hide my streaming tears, I tried to gain some semblance of composure before replying, "Then when you see Jesus, you can tell him you turned over every rock you could."

And that's when she uttered the words I never wanted to hear, "Michael...I want you to find love again."

At that moment, I could no longer contain myself, but somehow managed to choke out the words, "My sweet, darling Amanda...the ring stays on." Then all was still, and we simply held each other's hand until we got home.

Due to the extreme congestion on the highway, what was normally a five-hour trip turned into a torturous eight-and-a-half-hour ride. To say her exhaustion level was off the charts would be to make the greatest of understatements, and I was absolutely distraught that she had to spend so much extra time in the car.

During the 8 ½ hour drive home from San Diego (due to construction), we stopped at Coco's in Baker. We had come to view this oasis and its manager, Max, as a most welcome respite on the desperate and all-too-frequent ride, and went in there with some frequency due to their easy access bathrooms. However, on this particular occasion, as we were leaving, Max followed us back to the car. In his arms, he carried a huge platter of the most sumptuous strawberries either of us had ever seen. When he presented them to Amanda, my eyes welled with tears at the supreme generosity and kindness he showed to my rapidly failing wife. As he handed them over, he simply said, "You enjoy, sweetheart." The pureness of the love and compassion displayed through his gesture absolutely made me burst with happiness and gratitude that someone could so deeply touch her heart at that very moment in time. He was a seemingly ordinary man who became, and will always remain, an extraordinary hero in my eyes. And because it happened to be one of the only things Amanda could hold down by then, my gratitude was multiplied ten-fold as I watched her relish every single bite.

In Amanda's Words...

Lots going on lately, and it's become difficult for me to be on the computer for any length of time because of the tumor on my tailbone.

That was the last sentence Amanda ever wrote, and I had to finish it for her. It was April 8th.

Throughout our relationship, whenever an argument was about to ensue, I would pause at its beginning and say to Amanda, "I love you...I love you," repeating it as many times as it took to quell the impending storm. She would always do the same. That night, as I was filming with our camcorder, telling her how well she had done to finish her protein shake, she suddenly interrupted me midstream. Looking straight into the lens, she began to repeat our trademark phrase over and over. After five or so "I love you," I started to laugh with joy and gratitude, as I knew exactly what she was doing. My precious wife wanted to put it on film in an effort to ensure that I would never ever forget. As if that were possible...

The following morning, Murphy's Law was once again in full swing, and she even had problems trying to get started in the oxygen chamber. The device made her feel very claustrophobic, which only served to compound her pain and high anxiety. But ever the trooper—right up to the very end—she vowed to try it again the next day.

The tumor on the back of Amanda's right leg had become infected and was giving off a grotesque smell, so the homeopathic doctor and I tried to clean out the area using a solution of saline and a white cream. We then applied honey (known for its antiseptic and antioxidant properties) and wrapped it up. She was in more pain at this time than is seemingly possible for any human to endure, and yet continued to soldier on to the very best of her ability. The morphine just wasn't touching it any longer.

There was something going on with her thinking, and she wasn't responding the way she should have been. Reading was out of the question. I thought she needed to have an MRI done immediately to determine what was going on. Additionally, she had more tumors than I could count and cried out in pain constantly. Naturally she was running on sheer terror, and I've never felt more completely helpless and spent.

Kristi was staying with us at the time, and during one long extremely dark night, Amanda got out of bed and walked to the doorway of our room where Kristi greeted her. "Are you okay, Amanda? Do you need anything?" Kristi asked. My wife then started to cry. The paralyzing fear that etched her face took my breath away.

She stared right into her sister's eyes and said, with tears flowing down her face, "I'm so scared. Am I dying? God help me!" Instantly, Kristi began to weep as well as she held her sister with the purest love I have ever witnessed between siblings.

As soon as we laid Amanda back into bed, Kristi rushed out of the room. Obviously she needed to get some air or just cry. I lay down with Amanda and just held her. I remember after her saying, "God help me," a calm seemed to settle over her. And although her speech was then severely affected, I knew she could hear me because, when I told her I loved her, she immediately responded in kind, without a hint of hesitation in her voice. It's a moment that will live with me forever.

The next afternoon, something happened to her brain, and she could no longer have a conversation. I believe she understood us but couldn't respond. Her behavior so reminded me of my father's in the last stages of Alzheimer's that I was dumbstruck. I honestly couldn't believe this was happening and was in a total state of panic and shock.

As tears poured down my cheeks, I finally admitted to myself that Amanda was going home to the Lord. My most precious and brave wife was going to go to heaven. I didn't know if it was going to be that day or the next; I just understood that it was going to be very soon. Although we had an appointment the following morning to go and see a doctor for a possible MRI, I already knew that, once I got her down to Vegas, she'd never come home again. I also understood in my heart that she didn't want to leave this earth from a hospital room. But still, I was so torn. For a year and a half, we had done nothing but fight; however now, reluctantly, I was forced to face the fact that it was time to lay down our weapons and let her go. I didn't know any other way.

I prayed to God to please hold my wife in His loving arms and assure her that I will see her again. "Tell her my love for her will never diminish and fill her heart with joy. You know how much she has suffered. Please, please help me get through this. I need your help. Oh, God, please give me strength to go on."

Later that night as I was lying next to Amanda, she seemed to be sleeping in something of a strangely tranquil comfort. Nevertheless, her head was profusely sweating, and her feet were starting to swell. In addition, she remained largely unresponsive. You didn't have to be a doctor to understand that those signs weren't good.

However, as I was stretching her legs, she suddenly awoke and started to sit up. When we made eye contact, I immediately said, "I love you, Amanda." I then went to kiss her, and was totally stunned when she actually puckered her lips and kissed me back...twice! I will remember those last kisses for the rest of my life and am so grateful to my angelic wife for letting me know that, even as death hovered near, the light of her love could never be diminished.

In the Blink of an Eye

My mother-in-law and I were up most of that night. Around 12:30 a.m., Amanda had three grand mall seizures, which lasted about five minutes each. We thought the Lord was going to take her then, but she wasn't quite ready to give into the final defeat. However, her breathing was becoming increasingly shallow, and we knew the time was drawing near. It was Good Friday, and I couldn't think of a more appropriate day for her to meet her maker.

Her cats were all surrounding her and Tigger, her favorite, had been crying nonstop for three days; something he'd never done before or since that time.

I could still catch glimpses of consciousness when I called her name, but my heart was shattering into a million pieces. I was simply too exhausted to shed any more tears.

By early that evening, Amanda's breathing had become even more labored, and her heart rate was way too fast. The hospice worker said that if she had been an older person, she would have gone much sooner. The problem, you see, was that she was just too young to die. Other than the cancer, her body was still strong, and she was fighting to live right up until the bitter end.

When, just minutes later, Amanda began to once again convulse, I was on her right side, Kristi was on the left and her mother was at the head of our bed. As her arms flailed uncontrollably in the air and her body continued to violently seize, Connie straddled her dying child. With their fingers intertwined and legs pressed together, she whispered, "Mandy, my baby, you pushed your way out of me into this world; now push against me as you leave it."

After about five minutes, the seizure finally stopped. However, the damage was done, for Amanda could now only breathe from one side of her mouth.

Connie and I were both severely sleep deprived, as we had been up for days. So I laid down on one side of Amanda, with her mother on the other. I remember us saying that we would both try and sleep, but about two minutes later, we each peeked at the same time to see if the other had actually accomplished that impossible feat, causing us to both chuckle a tiny bit. We knew neither of us was going to get any rest because we wanted every second of time we could spend with Amanda.

At 2:07 p.m. on April 15, 2006, surrounded by all of those she held nearest and dearest to her heart, my beautiful wife, Amanda Faye Brown, passed on. She was thirty-one years old. I held her in my arms the whole time and, with two of her last three breaths, she murmured, "I love you, Michael…I love you Michael." With that, her breathing stopped. I whispered, "In the blink of an eye, I will be with you again…in the blink of an eye."

At the very instant she left us, the wind outside began to howl. It was as if God Himself had swept down and whisked her away on His wings. Her father, who was sitting in the corner, immediately said, "I feel so much peace in this room right now." And while I was stunned that he would make such a statement at that very moment, I've come to believe that the Lord was speaking through him in an effort to provide us with a small element of the comfort and reassurance we were so desperately seeking. For although I screamed out in the kind of gut-wrenching pain only one who has experienced such a loss can truly understand, I was grateful for His heavenly gift.

Amanda's grandfather, who died at Christmas later that year, was in our living room when Amanda passed away. I couldn't bear to allow the mortuary people to put the sheet over her head as they wheeled her out, and just before reaching the front door, he yelled, "STOP!" Rising from his chair, the elderly man walked over to Amanda, leaned down, and with a kiss to her forehead, simply said, "See ya later, kiddo," and then she was gone.

I can only continue to live my life as I believe she would have wanted me to. As such, I've dedicated it to honoring this wonderful woman through my work with the Melanoma Education Foundation. She's shining in heaven now; of this I am sure. For whenever I look up and see that special sparkle in the sky—even on the darkest of days—I'm certain it's my Amanda smiling at me once more.

Memories of Amanda

From Bob Sachs

Strength, courage, and a beautiful smile through adversity—that was Amanda Brown. Her determination and will to fight this terrible disease demonstrated to all that life can be tenuous, but her underlying message was always, "Never give up!"

I met Michael Brown in the fall of 2004. We were hired to play together at a new club opening at the Mandalay Bay Hotel. He is one of the most talented people I know. What a performer! He could play, sing, dance, and entertain like nobody's business. We got to be the *best* of friends. We always shared each other's ideas—different approaches to music: interpretation, feel, style, etc., but, the number one subject was always his wonderful wife, Amanda. A couple so in love…it was a perfect marriage. She was his biggest supporter. She was so proud of Michael. You certainly need that in this business. Amanda would sometimes come backstage and embrace everyone with her beautiful, radiant smile and this incredible zest for life. Then, the unthinkable happened—Amanda became sick. She was diagnosed with malignant melanoma.

I think back now of the year and a half they both fought this horrible disease. They tried everything: doctors, medications, chemotherapy, radiation, and blood transfusions. Time was just slipping away. Michael and

I spent a lot of time between shows just talking, trying to gather strength. On stage, he always played his ass off. No one ever knew what he was going through, except for the people who cared.

Amanda Brown lost her life on April 15, 2006. She was a person of great character. She was warm, affectionate, sincere, fun, and most of all, loving. My short friendship with her was quite special. She was someone that you always wanted to be around. I will never forget her. She has become a part of my life, and I will carry her smile and her legacy with me for the rest of my life.

From Barry and Susie Shade

Barry and I were introduced to Amanda by our close friend, "Downtown" Michael Brown. We were captivated by his flirtatious personality and exceptional talent as a saxophone musician. He has a heart of gold, and his soulful emotions are expressed through his music. We get a kick out of watching the effect he has on people in nightclubs. Just imagine an atmosphere of ordinary people just socializing, and then in the background you hear a few musical notes being played as if his sax was speaking to you. His meek stage presence lures people into listening while he continues to play and tease an audience. He plays a room like he is getting his inspirational music vibes from the crowd, and they start egging him on for more! Michael would intentionally hold back his professional capabilities and then just let it rip! What a thrill it is in watching him bring down the house. People would end up dancing everywhere, including tabletops and platforms. He never left a club without people thanking him for a good time or asking where he would be performing next.

There is no doubt that Michael received a lot of attention from women, but there was only one special lady that he wanted to introduce to us; her name was Amanda Faye Welton.

We were living in Huntington Beach and received a phone call from Michael. He said, "I'm bringing my future wife out to meet you, and I'm going to put her on the phone right now to talk to you." Amanda started talking with so much excitement in her voice. She said she looked forward to meeting us and couldn't wait to get to the beach to smell the ocean and put her feet in the sand. From that moment on, we could see what Michael saw in her.

The things in life that most of us take for granted were priceless moments for her. When Amanda arrived, she immediately hugged us like she had known us for years. She was an attractive redhead with a beautiful smile, and she made us feel comfortable right away. Amanda was like a breath of fresh air that couldn't help but make you feel young again. She was immensely proud of "her Michael" and often talked about how she was going to help him with his career. She just loved him so, and the feeling was, of course, completely mutual.

Barry and I quickly realized that Amanda was a bright, young businesswoman way beyond her years. She conveyed to us that she was going to create a website to expose Michael's talent for people to see all over the world. We had no idea she could build and design her own web page, but her actions spoke louder than words, and she managed to accomplish that, too!

Her website ended up being a huge success. Amanda consistently e-mailed family, friends, and fans of current events that were taking place in their lives, and she also managed to actually make video recordings of Michael's concert tours with well-known musicians.

As a couple, Michael and Amanda could light up a room and put a smile on your face no matter what else was going on around them. To know them truly is to love and adore them. This is why it became difficult for many loved ones to accept the health challenges that would tragically shorten their married life together.

It is extremely difficult to express your feeling to close loved ones when they are desperately reaching out for your help and you are witnessing the pain and suffering they endured together for the longest time. Reading their website and witnessing their unshakeable faith and hope for a miracle cure just ripped our hearts to pieces. Amanda's courage and fight for life were beyond anyone's imagination.

I sat down in my home office many times attempting to write a message in Amanda's web guest book and spent countless hours reading all the inspirational ones that were sent to her from around the world. Barry and I viewed pictures of Amanda's current health conditions from experimental cancer treatments in hospitals, then I would get this image in my mind of Michael's journey from one state to the next, sharing in Amanda's dream of finding a cure to end this battle.

The reality of what Michael managed to accomplish was overwhelming. He drove to and from the hospital in California constantly with no time to sleep; yet he continued to find the strength to go straight to work, convincing himself that "the show must go on." Whenever we'd ask him how he was holding up, he would simply reply, "Nothing I've done has even come close to what Amanda's going through."

By the time I finished reading and absorbing all of the information about the new treatment, I found myself mentally exhausted. I would just break down and cry with heartfelt frustration and anger. At the same time, my soul felt cleansed, and I knew that the Lord was working on my faith through Amanda!

The next day while feeling discouraged, I would find myself reaching out to coworkers and family members. I started sharing the story of how our friendship began and the challenges that Michael and Amanda were facing today.

I told them to click onto their website so they could see how beautiful she was and how she expressed herself. People started calling me, asking me to relay to the couple their sincerest sympathy. They would tell me that they had sent Amanda an inspirational message and could relate to her illness due to losing one of their own loved ones to cancer or an untimely death. These individuals were strangers compelled to return to her website daily. She shared her personal journal of what she was experiencing while capturing the hearts of many readers. It was like reading a rewrite to

"Love Story," feeling your heart ache while balling your eyes out.

On March 4, 2006, Barry and I received a phone call from Mike. He said the cancer was taking over Amanda's body, and we needed to come visit her now. When we arrived, Amanda was in extreme pain and discomfort. She was sitting upright in bed with her laptop on her thighs, and her main concern was fixing her website that was currently down. She was frustrated that she couldn't retrieve her inspirational messages and was anxious to update readers about her experience in Hawaii as well as how she was currently feeling. Amanda told me stories about people who replied to her from all over the world. These inspirational thoughts and prayers were priceless gifts of love to her.

Upon our arrival at their home, we were not prepared to see Amanda in her current condition. Barry and I had stopped going to the website prior to our visit because we could not bear to watch Amanda's beautiful body deteriorate, so it was quite a shock.

As soon as we hugged her and she felt our love, she made us laugh by just being her sweet, naive self! After the embrace, we could only see our beautiful Amanda, and she was talking like it was just another ordinary day!

We tried to be strong and kept busy doing what ever we could. Barry did yard work, and I started gathering her laundry to wash. Michael was consistently consoling her while praying out loud together.

She was emotionally distraught because she refused to accept that her body just wasn't allowing her to take care of personal needs. I told her that she was being way too hard on herself, and the doctors wanted her to rest and let other people help her! This was unthinkable for Amanda. I don't know how Michael kept his cool for so long without falling apart, but first and foremost in his mind was making sure that she had adequate medication to ease her pain.

I soon left the room and went out to the front yard where I discovered a man from the church removing debris. I asked him if he knew Amanda, and he replied no; the Lord had just sent him there to make her front yard beautiful. He said that he had once briefly spoken with her, and she had deeply touched his heart. Apparently Amanda had told him that her favorite flower was the Casa Blanca lily, and he said all he could think about was filling the whole yard with lilies so she could look out her front window and see the beautiful flowers. Michael soon joined me and asked the man why he was doing this. He replied, "I didn't want to miss out on a blessing." After absolutely insisting he accept one hundred dollars for the work, he asked Mike the same question, "Why are you doing this?"

Without skipping a beat, Michael replied in kind, "Because I don't want to miss out on a blessing, either."

This is the motivational impact Amanda would unknowingly have on people. She had a special gift in planting her own seeds of love.

I tried to think of a gift that I could give her at a time like this. I went back into her room and sat down next to her on the bed. I told her that she reminded me of the person that Pastor Rick teaches about in his book, "The Purpose Driven Life." It's about how to receive eternal life, and although Amanda said she had heard about the book, she'd never had the opportunity to read it. When I told her that she was an example of what Jesus had intended when he spoke about the way in which we all should live, she merely shrugged and said that she didn't think she had done anything special. I then reminded her of the multitudes of hearts she had touched through her website and also let her know that, because of her, I had renewed my faith. How I wish I could be more like her.

When Barry and I returned home, Amanda telephoned me, and I could hear from the sound of her voice that she was in good spirits. She conveyed to me that she had found the book to be very inspirational, and I couldn't have been happier to hear it.

I wanted Amanda to gracefully accept the quiet prayers of her loved one's wishes. She is now in the hands of our heavenly Father, and we just want her to have pleasant dreams of a new beginning in a beautiful, pain-free world!

We are so proud of Michael's endless faith and the love he continues to share with everyone. If anyone out there is still uncertain about what true love is, they'll know for certain after reading this book.

From Steven Day

The first time I met Amanda was in 1999. She was with one of my dearest, lifelong friends, Mike Brown, to whom I've remained so close that every time I phone him in Vegas from New York, we inevitably revert back to our adolescent behavior. It's always like the seventh grade all over again! If Amanda picked up the phone when I called, we'd exchanged pleasantries before she graciously handed him the phone. Always a good sport, I vividly remember hearing her laughing in the background as he was "rousting" me. She knew how ridiculous we were; yet, it seemed to amuse her as well. Most people, especially the wife of a childhood friend, would probably have thought we should have gotten past such antics, but she somehow seemed to understand the bond that propelled our behavior.

Sometimes I would receive a message on my phone from Amanda, and I was certain to hear Mike giggling in the background. He was obviously the instigator behind her "working me." But the timing never failed to be perfect, with the jovial spirit that emitted from the other end of the line making the obstacles of daily life seems so trivial and insignificant.

Of course it wasn't all frivolity with Amanda, and through our conversations, I acquired a better understanding of not only her career aspirations, but of her developing faith as well. I also came to fully realize the depth of her staunch support for Michael's talent as a professional musician. It gave me great comfort to know that he was with someone who nurtured and understood his many gifts so well.

Finally, at Michael's and my twenty-year high school reunion, I got a chance to meet Amanda in person. She was so happy to be there with Mike. I remember her smiling and hanging onto him all evening; I also noted how very proud she was of him. I felt like

I was meeting not just one old friend, but now two. A great beauty, I recall thinking how lucky my friend was to have found the love of his life.

Not long after that event, Mike notified me of her skin cancer and how quickly it had spread. One time when she came to LA to seek treatment, I happened to be out there visiting family for the Christmas holidays and was able to pick her up at the LA airport. My brother had also been able to find her housing near the hospital. In retrospect, I realize how fortunate I was to have been able to spend this time with her. We shopped and made dinners together, and my brother and I drove her to her appointments. During the course of our time together, she shared so many of her thoughts with me: about the illness, her love for Michael, and how much she believed in and supported his talent as a musician. We also discussed her newfound appreciation of the importance of consuming healthy foods, her passion for growing fruits and vegetables in her garden, and her optimism and willingness to try any new medical treatments she could find to beat the cancer that was rapidly eating her alive. However, what touched me most was how, in the middle of all the devastation she was going through, her faith never wavered.

As with all who were fortunate enough to get to know Amanda, I was the recipient of her enormous kindness and strength, enough to keep her spirit alive within me always.

From Jane Maclean Craig

Much to my extreme regret, I never had the great good fortune of meeting this truly phenomenal woman in life. However, in the process of chronicling her unbelievably heartbreaking and courageous journey, I have come to know a spirit absolutely like no other. She has affected me in ways too profound to express in the context of these few words, but let me just say, it has been one of the greatest honors of my life to help tell the world her story. The unparalleled love and devotion she and Michael shared is the stuff of legends and, together, they represent the very best humanity has to offer. God most certainly broke the mold the day He created Amanda Faye Brown, and she will live on in my heart and mind forever.

From the Author

Let me close by saying that my experience with Amanda's illness and incredibly premature passing was the most unbelievably gut-wrenching journey anyone could ever imagine taking. Through the heart breaking darkness and lingering pain since her loss, I have found light by fervently striving to honor her fondest wish: that I seek to educate as many as possible about the very real and completely preventable dangers that conspired to end her beautiful young life at the age of 31. As such, I have taken the position of Executive Director for the Nevada Chapter of the Melanoma Education Foundation. In this capacity, I have, with the sustenance of her memory, visited numerous middle and high schools throughout the state, where I spread the message of the life-saving importance of sun protection.

I couldn't possibly end this book without a personal tribute to the love of my life, Amanda Faye Brown, the phenomenal woman who inspired it. In spite of the agony we experienced in our relatively short time together, I thank God every night for affording me the extraordinary privilege of loving and being loved by the most courageous and unbelievably wonderful woman a man could be blessed to know. We truly had it all, and I consider myself an enormously lucky man for being the one to stand by her side.